W9-DGE-592

"A must-read! Louisa Grandin Sylvia's wellness plan addresses the key ingredients essential to creating a healthy lifestyle."

—**Muffy Walker, MSN, MBA**, cofounder and chairman of the International Bipolar Foundation

"When dealing with depression and other mood-related issues, we who have mood disorder diagnoses can become laser-focused on deficits or 'fixing' what's 'wrong.' While symptom reduction and elimination are naturally goals of most people's treatment plans, these can—and I'd say must—be joined with concurrent creation of wellness practices. Louisa Grandin Sylvia's book is an empowering road map for those of us who want to shift our focus from solely reaction to symptoms to proactive creation of resiliency-enhancing diet, exercise, sleep, and other wellness-related choices."

—**Allen Doederlein**, president of the Depression and Bipolar Support Alliance

"There is no easy solution to creating a healthier lifestyle, especially if you have bipolar disorder, but this book can help. It offers user-friendly tools to increase your motivation to make the necessary lifestyle changes that you need to improve your mental and physical health. Anyone living with mood disturbance could benefit from reading this book."

—**Lauren B. Alloy, PhD**, professor at Joseph Wolpe Distinguished Faculty and director of clinical training at Temple University in Philadelphia, PA

"Louisa Grandin Sylvia has assembled an extraordinary resource that succinctly and comprehensively brings together empirically supported science and recommendations to preserve and regain health. I would strongly recommend that this book, written in an accessible manner, be on the reading list of any individual who strives for optimal physical and mental health."

—**Roger S. McIntyre, MD, FRCPC**, professor of psychiatry and pharmacology at the University of Toronto, and head of the Mood Disorders Psychopharmacology Unit at the University Health Network

"We have only recently understood that lifestyle factors including smoking, physical inactivity, and poor diet contribute to a person's risk of developing mood problems. We now know that addressing these factors reduces symptoms in people who have mood problems. What's missing is a practical synthesis of this information to guide people who have mood problems on how to target these factors to improve their physical and mental health. This book by Louisa Grandin Sylvia, an acknowledged expert in lifestyle and mood disorders, is an invaluable aid for those wishing to take control of their lifestyles and improve their mood."

—**Michael Berk, MD, NHMRC**, senior principal research fellow and Alfred Deakin Professor of Psychiatry at the Deakin University School of Medicine

"Despite decades of research, there is no silver bullet that will quickly end bipolar disorder. The best way for someone with bipolar disorder to reclaim their life is by crafting a health-promoting lifestyle. The research on the effects of sleep, diet, and exercise are each compelling. This book brings the pieces together into an integrated approach that is clearly explained, with examples based on stories of people who have succeeded, and based on ongoing research. Experts advocate a lifestyle approach for 'heart health.' Louisa Grandin Sylvia provides a plan for 'brain health.' The strategies will complement other treatments by focusing on quality of life, energy, and functioning, not just reducing the symptoms and stress associated with bipolar disorder. This book is a leading example of the next-generation approach to mood disorders, recognizing the connection between body and mind and using that to help the whole person."

—**Eric Youngstrom, PhD**, professor of psychology and psychiatry at the University of North Carolina at Chapel Hill

"In this important book, Louisa Grandin Sylvia provides readers with a step-by-step approach for improving diet, exercise, and sleep—all habits that can have powerful effects on mood and health. Readers will find this book rich in information and clinical examples, with crucial attention devoted to the barriers and bad habits that can derail wellness goals."

—**Michael W. Otto, PhD**, professor of psychological and brain sciences at Boston University and author of *Exercise for Mood and Anxiety Disorders*

The
Wellness
Workbook
for
Bipolar Disorder

Your Guide to Getting Healthy
& Improving Your Mood

LOUISA GRANDIN SYLVIA, PhD

New Harbinger Publications, Inc.

Jefferson Twp Library
1031 Weldon Road
Oak Ridge, N.J. 07438
973-208-6244
www.jeffersonlibrary.net

Publisher's Note

This publication is designed to provide accurate and authoritative information in regard to the subject matter covered. It is sold with the understanding that the publisher is not engaged in rendering psychological, financial, legal, or other professional services. If expert assistance or counseling is needed, the services of a competent professional should be sought.

Distributed in Canada by Raincoast Books

Copyright © 2015 by Louisa Grandin Sylvia
        New Harbinger Publications, Inc.
        5674 Shattuck Avenue
        Oakland, CA 94609
        www.newharbinger.com

Cover design by Amy Shoup
Acquired by Catharine Meyers
Edited by Jasmine Star

All Rights Reserved

Library of Congress Cataloging-in-Publication Data

Sylvia, Louisa Grandin.
  The wellness workbook for bipolar disorder : improve your mood, lose weight, and feel better / Louisa Grandin Sylvia, PhD.
    pages cm
  Includes bibliographical references.
  ISBN 978-1-62625-130-4 (paperback) -- ISBN 978-1-62625-131-1 (pdf e-book) -- ISBN 978-1-62625-132-8 (epub) 1. Manic-depressive illness. 2. Manic-depressive illness--Treatment. 3. Manic-depressive illness--Nutritional aspects. 4. Behavior modification. 5. Self-care, Health. I. Title.
  RC516.S95 2015
  616.89'5--dc23

               2015005421

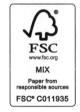
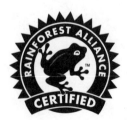

Printed in the United States of America

17   16   15

10 9 8 7 6 5 4 3 2 1   First printing

For my clients, whose stories are the backdrop to this book.
You have taught me so much.

For my family, who have had the patience and fortitude to stick by me.
You covered for me every step of the way.

Thank you.

Contents

Foreword

Creating a healthy lifestyle starts something that can be described as a memory of the future (Ingvar 1985). By having a memory of the future—keeping in mind your ultimate goals—you can get to a healthier lifestyle. But getting there is often more challenging than any of us would like, especially for those with bipolar disorder. Who wouldn't like to lose five or ten pounds? Who wouldn't like to exercise more because it's so good for a person's health? Who wouldn't like to get the right amount of sleep, drink a little less, and, for those who take recreational drugs, try to cut down or stop? We get stuck in habits and find it difficult to change those habits by ourselves, even when we know better. What we need is a good coach. Lucky for you, you got one when you picked up this book.

Amidst the burdens of bipolar disorder, healthy living tends to take a backseat to mood episodes of depression, mania, or hypomania. But isn't being healthy or well just what you want? It's not good enough to simply be free of mood episodes and symptoms. Wellness is not just the absence of these symptoms; it's so much more—feeling that you're a part of something larger, having a sense of personal growth, having relationships that are mutually satisfying, feeling that you're the author of your own life and that you're approaching that task with a sense of competence and mastery, and feeling good about who you are (Ryff 2014). These goals are challenging enough for people who don't have bipolar disorder, and even more challenging for those who do. To achieve this kind of wellness you have to go on a journey. And on any difficult journey, you need a guide. This book can be that guide.

The ways you behave, the choices you make, and what you ultimately do all determine your lifestyle. The ways you behave depend on the ways you think, the choices you make depend on the ways you think, and the decisions you make depend on the ways you think. In fact, the *ways you think* depend on the ways you think. This book will give you new ways to think about wellness to ease the process of changing what you do to live more in alignment with your wellness goals.

You can achieve wellness by taking small, gradual steps toward a healthy lifestyle. Eat a little better and then continue to improve what you eat. Exercise a little more and then turn that into a habit. Learn to think about the future impacts of your decisions and try to become a little less impulsive, considering whether your decisions bring you closer to or further from your goals and values. Then you can make that a habit too. Yet even these modest goals can seem overwhelming. Dr. Sylvia and her book are here to help you.

Ultimately, achieving wellness has to be doable. It may take some time, as you break your big, overall goals down to smaller, realistic goals. Dr. Sylvia's methods will help you stick with the program. Let's say you want to lose a few pounds. By cutting out the equivalent of a teaspoon of sugar a day (about 100 calories) from your diet, in six months you can lose five pounds. Sounds easy, right? But if it were, everyone would do that, and no one would struggle with being overweight. The trick, and the foundation of this book, is to make the ultimate goal not to lose weight, but to live a healthier lifestyle. By doing so, you can not only lose weight, but also feel better and more energetic and be healthier overall. Dr. Sylvia will give you the tools for doing this.

On your journey toward wellness and a healthier you, you may find that you sometimes turn into a harsh coach, giving yourself a hard time when you get off track, which can lead to feeling like you're a failure or wanting to give up. You might tell yourself that it doesn't matter and you might as well eat that entire pint of ice cream because you can't lose weight anyway. This book can help you look at these kinds of thoughts and make better decisions, in part by being kinder and more forgiving to yourself.

Finally, by having a healthier lifestyle, you can also improve your bipolar disorder. Eating well, exercising regularly, sleeping better, and making healthier choices are all good for your brain. Stick with the program, be kind to yourself, and have a great journey to wellness.

—Andrew A. Nierenberg, MD

Acknowledgments

I have learned that no one ever writes a book alone, even if she or he is the sole author. I wish that I could list thirty, or maybe sixty, coauthors, because so many people have helped shape this book. The following is a short (and not exhaustive) list of those that I would like to thank for helping me.

To my clients: Thank you for telling me your stories and trusting enough to share the deepest, darkest, scariest parts of these stories with me. You've taught me many things, but most importantly for this book, that it truly isn't easy to make lifestyle changes when you live with the thoughts and feelings so common in bipolar disorder. I've tried to really listen and put what you've done and the positive changes you've made in these pages to give hope to others by sharing what has helped you succeed.

To my mentors and colleagues: Many of the ideas and skills taught in this book have been shaped by talking to you. There are many people who have taught me things, but there are two mentors I must mention individually. Andrew Nierenberg, MD, has been a tireless supporter of my work, and through his innovation and clarity of thought, he has greatly improved the treatment and care of people with mood disorders. He has taught me to be persistent and thoughtful and, perhaps most importantly (as it can be rare in academic medicine), to have fun. Lauren Alloy, PhD, is entirely responsible for helping me to get from the idea of being a clinical researcher to actually being one. She stuck by me, wrote many, many letters of support, and always said, "You can do it, Louisa." Thank you.

To my family: I have been blessed to have the most supportive and caring family. My parents were certainly the first people who told me, "You can do it." I've come to recognize how important that message is in my life, given that so many things seem scary until you actually start doing them. One of the best things about my parents is that they stand by me even when I don't do things very well. This is a true sign of unconditional love, and it's amazing stuff. My brothers aren't so bad either. They have been, and always will be, my go-to guys when the going gets tough. My mother-in-law has proven to be my secret weapon. While I am away at work, writing late at night, or sitting in some conference, she maintains the home front and makes sure that my kids are well fed, have clean clothes, and are getting a whole bunch of love. My kids are still very little people right now, but they completely ground me and remind me that they are the most important things going on in my life, always. My role as a mother will always be my first commitment. I love you guys.

To my husband: You have somehow managed to be my best friend, confidant, coworker, coparent, and so many other roles, all rolled up into one person. I'm not sure how you find the flexibility to be so many different things for me, but I am so thankful that you continue to find a way to do this as our lives get more challenging and complicated. In short, this book, and so many other things, would not happen without your support. You are my true partner.

To my friends: I joke with you that I haven't made a new friend in almost a decade. Thanks for being my buddies through all of these years.

Finally, my publisher paired me up with an incredible editor. I am so thankful for this, as she has shaped this book to be clearer, more organized, and hopefully just a better tool for everyone who picks it up. Thanks, Jasmine.

To all the readers of this book, let me leave you with my favorite line: "You can do it!" I really think you can. You can make these lifestyle changes. I believe in you. No one is perfect. We all struggle, and people with bipolar disorder will struggle more than most, but you can do it.

Introduction

This book is designed to help people with bipolar disorder create a healthier lifestyle. This is important, as many people with bipolar disorder don't seem to feel better, or well enough, when just taking their medications. In fact, more than 50 percent of people with bipolar disorder who are taking medications still report having uncomfortable or bothersome symptoms (Keitner et al. 1996). For this reason, it's a good idea for people with bipolar disorder to consider being in therapy in addition to taking medications. The best treatment for bipolar disorder consists of taking medications and being in therapy (Huxley, Parikh, and Baldessarini 2000; Yatham et al. 2005).

I am a psychologist and therefore an expert in therapy, but not in prescribing medications. This book is based on my work in developing a particular therapy to help people with bipolar disorder feel better, but I also believe that medications are an important part of treating bipolar disorder. For this reason, I suggest that you consider using this book while seeing someone to prescribe medications for your bipolar disorder, or that you at least see someone to discuss this option.

In regard to therapy, there are many different types. You may have heard of cognitive behavioral therapy (A. T. Beck et al. 1979), or dialectical behavior therapy (Linehan 1993), or yet another kind of therapy. Many of these therapies are very useful in managing bipolar disorder. This book is based on research I've done in order to develop a therapy to help people with bipolar disorder create healthier lifestyles (Sylvia et al. 2011; Sylvia, Salcedo, et al. 2013). This therapy is called nutrition, exercise, and wellness treatment (NEW Tx), and this book covers topics in those three areas:

- **Nutrition**, or making healthy food choices and eating in moderation

- **Exercise**, and strategies to help you make exercise part of your weekly routine

- **Wellness**, which encompasses other key aspects of creating a healthy lifestyle, such as overcoming obstacles to a healthy sleep schedule, reducing use of substances, and increasing the likelihood of meeting and keeping friends

In short, the goal of this book is to help you create a healthier lifestyle so that you can ease your bipolar symptoms and improve your physical health and, in the process, feel better.

Is This a Diet Book?

People often ask me whether NEW Tx will help people with bipolar disorder lose weight. The answer is yes. However, this isn't the focus of the treatment, and therefore isn't the focus of this book. The aim of this book is to help you make changes to your life that are consistent with recommendations for how people with bipolar disorder can lead a healthier lifestyle. This often involves losing weight, but there are many other aspects of creating a healthy lifestyle that don't require losing weight. Therefore, I often caution people to not become overly focused on weight loss, as this is only one potential outcome of working with this program. Other potential outcomes include having fewer mood shifts, experiencing fewer or less intense depressive or manic symptoms, having better quality of life, enjoying more social support, improving your physical health, reducing the use of substances, and getting better sleep. That said, if weight loss is one of your personal goals, you'll certainly find skills to help you lose weight in this book.

How to Use This Book

As mentioned, this book is based on my work in developing NEW Tx, a form of therapy designed to help people with bipolar disorder lead healthier lifestyles. NEW Tx consists of eighteen sessions over twenty weeks and involves working with a therapist. Therefore, I strongly encourage you to seek support when using this book. Making changes to exercise habits, diet, and other aspects of your lifestyle can be challenging for anyone. It's difficult to break old habits and forge new patterns. (To further aid you in making difficult changes, in chapter 10 I'll address how to increase and maintain social support.)

You don't have to read the book straight through. I do, however, recommend that you read chapters 1 and 2 before any others, as they will help you effectively use the material in later chapters. For example, in chapter 2, you'll identify your goals for creating a more healthy lifestyle, along with intermediate goals for getting there, and this will be very useful in your work in later chapters. After reading chapters 1 and 2, it's fine to skip to the chapters that you feel will help you most. If sleep is your biggest challenge, you can skip to chapter 8 next. Or if you have difficulty with motivating yourself to change and think rewarding yourself may help you stick to a healthy lifestyle plan, read chapter 7 first. Some skills do build from chapter to chapter, but in those cases I'll refer back to earlier chapters covering a skill so you can read up on it and understand the foundation.

However, do be sure that you eventually read all of the chapters, as each has unique material that may be helpful for you even if the subject of that chapter isn't an issue for you. For example, in chapter 8, on sleep, I explain an extremely helpful problem-solving tool: a chain analysis. This approach can be used for any problem behavior, so you'll want to read chapter 8 at some point, even if sleep isn't a problem for you.

Based on my experiences in leading groups and treating individuals, I've found that everyone's needs are different. No two people have the same wellness goals, and I haven't found a "one size fits all" approach that works. This is particularly true for people with bipolar disorder. Instead, if you are to be successful in creating a healthy lifestyle, you need to understand your specific obstacles (identified by doing a behavior analysis) and then identify which specific skills will help you overcome them. This book will help you do all of that, and more. So let's get started!

Chapter 1

Getting Ready for Change

As mentioned in the introduction, this book is designed to help you create a healthier lifestyle. This is a worthwhile goal for anyone, but it's especially important for people with bipolar disorder because many elements of a healthy lifestyle, such as eating nutritiously, getting enough activity, and sleeping well, can ease bipolar symptoms. In this chapter, I'll give just a brief overview of bipolar disorder and some of the reasons why adopting a healthier lifestyle is in your best interest. Then we'll dive right in by looking at the process of change, determining whether you're ready to make changes, and starting to address any obstacles to change.

Types of Bipolar Disorder

There are two types of bipolar disorder. *Bipolar I disorder* is characterized by manic episodes: periods of abnormally elevated or high mood that last for at least seven days, with at least three of the following symptoms (American Psychiatric Association 2013):

- Having excessively high self-esteem or grandiose thoughts, such as *I am better than others*

- Having a decreased need for sleep or feeling rested with less sleep than usual

- Being more talkative than usual or exhibiting pressured speech, meaning being difficult to interrupt

- Having racing thoughts, with ideas flitting through the mind in quick succession, and becoming preoccupied with these thoughts

- Being easily distracted, with attention being captured by unimportant or irrelevant things

- Showing an increase in goal-directed activity, with a relentless drive to do or accomplish things, or excessive restlessness

- Overindulging in enjoyable behaviors with a high risk of negative outcomes, such as shopping sprees, risky sexual adventures, or improbable business schemes

Manic episodes may also be characterized by extreme irritability, in which case four of the above symptoms are necessary for a diagnosis of bipolar I. People with bipolar I disorder may also experience depression or *mixed episodes* (a combination of manic and depressive symptoms); however, a manic episode that impairs a person's ability to function is required for a diagnosis of bipolar I.

Bipolar II disorder is characterized by major depression, or lack of interest or sad mood for at least two weeks, plus five of the following symptoms (American Psychiatric Association 2013):

- Weight loss that isn't due to trying to diet, or weight gain

- Oversleeping or having trouble sleeping

- Experiencing psychomotor agitation, or restlessness, that is observable by others

- Feeling very tired or experiencing a loss of energy

- Feeling worthless or having inappropriate guilt, such as believing that you deserve to be punished in some way

- Having difficulty concentrating or making decisions

- Having recurrent thoughts of death, believing that life isn't worth living, or making a suicide attempt

People with bipolar II disorder may also experience less severe manic episodes, or *hypomania*. Like mania, hypomania is characterized by abnormally elevated or high mood or extreme irritability, but it's shorter in duration, lasting less than one week, and often it doesn't make it more difficult to function or otherwise interfere with a person's work, social life, or family life.

If you're unsure which type of bipolar disorder you have, this book on creating a healthier lifestyle will still be useful to you. I mention these subtypes because treatments often vary depending on the specific type of bipolar disorder, but not in this case. Thus, throughout this book, when I refer to "bipolar disorder," I'm referring to both bipolar I and bipolar II.

How Bipolar Disorder Can Affect Health

Recent evidence has raised the concern that people with bipolar disorder are at greater risk for developing cardiovascular disease or risk factors for cardiovascular disease, such as high blood pressure or diabetes, than people without bipolar disorder. Moreover, this risk of physical health complications among people with bipolar disorder appears to be increasing, perhaps due to the side effects of some medications used to treat the disorder, and also due to poor lifestyle choices (Kupfer 2005; Soreca, Frank, and Kupfer 2009). You may have noticed that it's harder to make healthy lifestyle choices when you don't feel well. This is common and affects people in many ways. For example, people who have bipolar disorder tend to eat fewer than two meals per day and consume more carbohydrates and sugar. They also report having difficulty buying or cooking food. This increases the likelihood of consuming unhealthy prepackaged or prepared foods and helps explain why people with mood disorders tend to be deficient in vitamins, minerals, and omega-3 fatty acids (Kilbourne et al. 2007).

For these reasons, researchers, myself included, are increasingly focused on the *physical* health of people with bipolar disorder. We want to improve the treatment of bipolar disorder by including lifestyle approaches, especially because physical complications can make bipolar disorder worse. For example, obesity, high blood pressure, and diabetes may be linked with depressive and manic episodes and psychiatric hospitalizations (Fagiolini et al. 2008); they also complicate the treatment and course of bipolar disorder (Angst et al. 2002). Hypothyroidism, obesity, and diabetes, which all occur more often among people with bipolar disorder, make it more difficult for people with bipolar disorder to function well and are associated with having more bipolar symptoms (Hirschfeld and Vornik 2005).

Now for the good news: Creating a healthier lifestyle will not only improve your physical health (weight, blood pressure, cholesterol, and so on), but will also help ease your symptoms of bipolar disorder. For example, one study found that, among people taking an antipsychotic medication commonly used in treating bipolar disorder (Olanzapine), a three-month educational program helped participants lose weight, and they also enjoyed increased quality of life, improved health, and a better body image (Evans, Newton, and Higgins 2005).

There's even more evidence that exercise can be very beneficial for mental health, in addition to physical health. One study found that exercising three days per week for forty-five minutes over a four-month period was as effective in reducing depressive symptoms as an antidepressant medication for people with unipolar depression (Blumenthal et al. 1999). It seems quite likely that exercise can be just as powerful for bipolar disorder, with one study showing that participating in a walking group five days per week for forty minutes helped decrease depression and anxiety symptoms among people with bipolar disorder (Ng, Dodd, and Berk 2007). In my studies, I've seen that when people with bipolar disorder increase their exercise, they report feeling much better (Sylvia, Salcedo, et al. 2013). This seems to apply to both subtypes of bipolar disorder: bipolar I and bipolar II.

Turning Things Around

To make the benefits of adopting a healthier lifestyle more concrete, let's look at an example of someone with bipolar disorder who made changes to her lifestyle and saw benefits in both her mental and physical health.

> Debra is a sixty-four-year-old college professor who often felt tired, unmotivated, and sad and wanted to be alone. She found it very difficult to get to class and often became short and irritable with her students when she was experiencing these symptoms of depression. During those times, Debra often slept fourteen to sixteen hours a day and reported that she had little or no appetite, though sometimes she treated herself to a large meal at her favorite Italian restaurant. Two to three times per year, Debra experienced several weeks of feeling extremely good. During these times, she felt unusually happy, was much more productive and talkative than usual, and needed less sleep, often just five or six hours per night. She noticed that she tended to have these elevated, or hypomanic, episodes when she went on trips, during which she tended to drink more alcohol and stay up later.

Debra wondered if her lifestyle was contributing to her overall feelings of not being well. She considered her tendency to oversleep, eat poorly, and avoid physical activity when she was depressed, and also her drinking and short hours of sleep when she was hypomanic. To test this theory, she started to make a point of scheduling more physical activity into her day during times when she was depressed, such as walking and horseback riding. She also resisted the urge to "treat herself," so instead of eating out, she cooked healthy meals at home. She also decided to travel less in order to reduce her tendency to drink, and also to keep from disrupting her daily routine, especially her sleep schedule. After several weeks, Debra began to feel more even-keeled. And as she took more control of her lifestyle, she noticed that her physical health was improving too. She was pleased that she had lost some weight and that her blood pressure was lower.

Debra's experience isn't uncommon. Research suggests that when people with bipolar disorder make healthier lifestyle choices, they experience both improvements in bipolar symptoms and a decrease in risk factors for cardiovascular disease (Kilbourne et al. 2008; Sylvia, Salcedo, et al. 2013).

Are You Ready to Change?

Who wouldn't want to have a healthier lifestyle, to lose weight and feel better? You may have already discovered that, unfortunately, wanting something doesn't mean you'll actually get it. For example, have you tried to diet before and been unsuccessful? Have you joined a gym in the hopes of exercising more only to have difficulty motivating yourself to go? My guess is that you've had these experiences, which are also common among people who don't have bipolar disorder. I believe that these difficulties aren't due to not wanting to change your diet and exercise routine; more likely, they're caused by other things getting in the way. Therefore, throughout this book we'll explore common obstacles to following through with making changes to adopt a healthier lifestyle. However, this won't help you unless you're truly ready to change.

So, how do you know when you're ready to change? You may have heard of the stages of change model, which describes the way many people go through the process of changing (Prochaska, Norcross, and DiClemente 1994). The following table describes the six stages of change and gives examples of each stage.

Stages of Change

Stage	Description	Example
Precontemplation	Having no intention of changing behavior and often denying that change is needed or believing oneself to be incapable of changing	"I don't need to exercise more." "Changing my diet won't help me." "I don't think that I'll be able to exercise regularly."
Contemplation	Acknowledging that change may be helpful, with vague plans to change, but not actually making any changes	"I should exercise more. Maybe I could join a gym." "I'd like to eat better, but changing my diet would be very hard."
Preparation	Being committed to making changes and making plans to change, with change likely to happen in the next month	"On January 1, I'll join the gym and start playing tennis." "Next month, I'll begin to monitor my food consumption to improve my portion control."
Action	Taking steps to actually change a behavior	"I'm going to the gym two times per week." "I only eat dessert three nights per week, as opposed to every night."
Maintenance	Continuing to maintain changes to prevent relapse	"I'm continuing to go to the gym and eat desserts in moderation."
Termination	No further effort is needed to maintain changes	"I enjoy going to the gym and eating healthier, and I no longer struggle with cravings for unhealthy foods."

Given that you've picked up this book and made it through the first few pages, it's likely that you're at least in the contemplation stage and have some vague plans to change. Perhaps you've already started committing to making healthy changes in your life and making plans to do so (the preparation stage). Or maybe you've already taken some steps to actually change your behavior (the action stage). It's also possible that you're in the maintenance stage or just looking for some extra tips to help you stay on track with a healthy lifestyle. This book can be helpful if you're in any of these stages. However, people often get stuck for years in the contemplation stage and have trouble moving from making vague plans to actually making changes. Consider Paul's story.

Paul likes to travel. He plans trips with his friends every few months, and he looks forward to going. He tends to spend about a week preparing for each trip: planning activities, buying things he needs for the trip, packing, and so on. His mood becomes quite elevated before and during these trips and he tends to need less sleep—sometimes only four hours per night. In contrast, when he gets back home, his mood becomes quite depressed and he usually sleeps more than twelve hours per night. Paul has been monitoring his mood for years, so he's well aware of his pattern of being hypomanic before and during his trips and depressed afterward. Paul has wanted to change his situation so that he doesn't experience so many ups and downs in mood, but he continues to travel and approach his trips in the same way.

What stage of change is Paul in? He recognizes that he needs to change in order to improve his mood and sleep, and he suspects that he may need to change his travel habits. Therefore he's no longer in the precontemplation stage. Yet Paul has made no plans or attempts to change his approach to travel or his sleep schedule, so he isn't yet in the preparation stage. Paul is stuck in the contemplation stage, recognizing the need to change and the potential benefits of doing so, but he hasn't taken any steps toward actually changing.

If you're stuck in the contemplation stage, becoming aware of this is the first key step. Imagine trying to take action while in the contemplation stage. You probably wouldn't be successful in making changes, and this could be very frustrating. This frustration can heighten negative thoughts about your ability to make changes (for example, *I'll never be able to lose weight*, *Exercise is too hard for me*, or *I crave unhealthy foods too much*). These thoughts, in turn, can make it even more challenging to move out of the contemplation stage. Therefore, recognizing that you're in the contemplation stage is the first step in making a change.

Behavior Analysis

The next step is to analyze your particular obstacles to making a certain change. One way of doing this is to pick a time in the past week when you didn't follow through on a change you wanted to make, such as not eating dessert after dinner. Then think of all the possible factors that might have contributed to eating dessert that night. These factors can include events, thoughts, feelings, and behaviors, even from the day before. This process of closely examining a behavior that you want to change and the related obstacles is called a *behavior analysis*.

I'll help you do your own behavior analysis shortly. But first, to give you a better idea of how it works, here's a sample worksheet that shows a completed behavior analysis for Karen, who ate dessert despite her plan not to.

Karen's Behavior Analysis Worksheet

Behavior to change: *Eating dessert after dinner on Wednesday night*	
When?	**Events, thoughts, feelings, and behaviors leading to the problem behavior**
Tues. 4 p.m.	*A friend at work was fired.*
Tues. 8 p.m.	*I chose not to have a dessert after dinner.*
Wed. 9 a.m.	*My friend wasn't at work today.*
Wed. 9 a.m.	*I missed my friend, and as a result, I felt sad.*
Wed. 10 a.m.	*I thought that I could be fired next, which made me feel unhappy, sad, and fearful.*
Wed. 12:30 p.m.	*I ate lunch alone and felt lonely.*
Wed. 3 p.m.	*I had two doughnuts for a snack, and then I felt guilty.*
Wed. 3:30 p.m.	*I had the thought that I'll never be able to eat healthy or manage my cravings for food, which makes me feel sad, disappointed, and angry.*
Wed. 5 p.m.	*I chose not to go for a walk after work.*
Wed. 6 p.m.	*I had the thought that I'll never be able to be healthy, which makes me feel sad.*
Wed. 7 p.m.	*I had the thought that it doesn't matter what I have for dinner because I already overate today, so now I'm frustrated.*
Wed. 7 p.m.	*I'm angry because I believe I'll never be able to lose weight.*
Wed. 8 p.m.	*I ate dessert.*

In that sample worksheet, you can begin to see some of the thoughts, feelings, and behaviors that led Karen to eat dessert on Wednesday night. Among other things, she was engaging in *emotional eating*, consuming unhealthy foods as a way to deal with negative emotions. The sample worksheet shows that Karen had negative emotions (sadness, fear), triggered by her friend being fired on Tuesday. You can also see how this stress led Karen to engage in other unhealthy behaviors, such as eating other unhealthy foods (doughnuts) and not exercising.

Exercise: Doing a Behavior Analysis

Now it's your turn to do your own behavior analysis. A blank worksheet for this purpose is provided here; a downloadable version of this worksheet is also available at http://www .newharbinger.com/31304. (See the back of the book for instructions on how to access it.) The downloadable version will come in handy for doing a behavior analysis for other problem behaviors in the future.

Take a minute to think of a behavior you'd like to change. It may be the reason you picked up this book—perhaps overeating, not exercising, drinking too much caffeine, or not sleeping well. Next, think of a very specific time in the past week when you engaged in this behavior that you'd like to change. For example, maybe you wanted to get to bed earlier on Friday night but instead stayed up until 2 a.m. In the following worksheet, write this behavior in the top row.

Next, spend some time carefully thinking about all of the thoughts, feelings, and behaviors (things you did) in the twenty-four hours leading up to when you engaged in this behavior that you'd like to change. If you have difficulty thinking of events, thoughts, feelings, and other behaviors that occurred before the problem behavior, ask a supportive family member or friend if he or she has noticed what typically happens before you engage the behavior.

Don't be tempted to skip over this exercise. Clearly identifying the problem behaviors that you want to change and knowing what triggers lead you to do them will be very useful as you work on setting goals for lifestyle changes in chapter 2. It will also help you choose strategies for creating a healthier lifestyle in the rest of the book.

The final step in moving out of the contemplation stage is identifying ways to manage potential triggers and other obstacles that you identify through behavior analysis. This book will be very helpful in this regard. It's full of techniques for changing thoughts, feelings, and behaviors. Each chapter will present at least one strategy to assist you in changing your behaviors so that you can be more successful in leading a healthier lifestyle.

Behavior Analysis Worksheet

Behavior to change:	
When?	**Events, thoughts, feelings, and behaviors leading to the problem behavior**

Keeping Your Bipolar Disorder in Mind

This book is different from other wellness books or diet and exercise books because it's geared specifically for people like you—people with bipolar disorder. Some skills that are helpful for people without bipolar disorder will also be helpful for you. For example, a basic and very important thing to do if you're trying to eat better is to monitor the foods you eat. This holds true regardless of whether you have bipolar disorder or not. However, if you have a mood disorder, how you monitor your diet, and also how you motivate yourself to do this, can differ. Thus, this book combines key strategies that have proven helpful for people in general with special modifications or skills for people with bipolar disorder. To give you an idea, here are some of the approaches specific to bipolar disorder covered in this book:

- Skills for challenging negative thoughts that make it difficult to adopt a healthier lifestyle—which should be helpful, given that people with bipolar disorder tend to have more frequent and intense negative thoughts

- Very concrete, specific advice on how you can make healthy changes, which is important because people with bipolar disorder often have difficulty with motivation

- Skills specific to emotional eating, or the tendency to eat as a way to manage uncomfortable mood, which is common among people with bipolar disorder

- Discussion of obstacles to acquiring the skills in this book that arise from bipolar disorder (such as mood shifts), as well as ways to overcome these obstacles

- Discussion of why certain skills may not be as helpful for people with bipolar disorder and how to adjust these skills so they can be more useful to you

Many of these considerations and modifications specific to people with bipolar disorder rely on techniques rooted in cognitive behavioral therapy, or CBT (Greenberger and Padesky 1995; J. S. Beck 2011). CBT skills are often designed to change behaviors and thoughts that aren't working for people in the hopes of making their lives better. The approach in this book incorporates many CBT skills that can assist you in making changes to your lifestyle.

Summary

- People with bipolar disorder tend to have unhealthy lifestyles.

- Creating a healthier lifestyle can improve your mental and physical health.

- There are different stages in the process of making changes.

- People often become stuck in the contemplation stage, not actually making changes.

- The first step to getting out of the contemplation stage is to be aware that this is your current stage of change.

- Conducting a behavior analysis can help you break out of the contemplation stage.

Chapter 2

Setting Goals

Things rarely "just happen," especially things that are difficult to do, such as adopting a healthier lifestyle. Therefore, this chapter will help you set concrete, specific goals for becoming healthier.

This chapter also focuses on setting realistic goals, as this will increase your likelihood of success. It's crucial that your plans for change be feasible, because if you have difficulty accomplishing your goals, you might believe you've failed—a belief that may make you give up on trying to change. This can be especially true for people with bipolar disorder, who tend to think more negatively (Scott et al. 2000; Alloy et al. 2006). In fact, it's common for people with bipolar disorder to think they've failed even when they're doing things successfully. Let's consider an example.

> Sarah, who has bipolar disorder, is in her midfifties and is unemployed. She lives alone with the exception of her dog, Sam. To cope with her down moods, Sarah sometimes drinks a beer in the evening or snacks on unhealthy foods. About ten years ago, she lost about twenty pounds due to making changes in her diet and exercise habits, but since then she's gained that weight back, along with an additional twenty pounds— something she monitors daily by weighing herself. Sarah has therefore developed the belief that she failed at dieting and exercising and is unlikely to be successful at either in the future.

Sarah is a client of mine, and when I met her, I realized that she'd made many changes on her own to adopt a healthier lifestyle. For example, over the years she's cut back on drinking considerably, and she attends support groups to help her live a sober life. She also walks Sam every day and often twice a day, and every once in a while she goes to the swimming pool to swim or walk in the water for strength training. Sarah also monitors what she eats and was therefore aware of eating patterns that weren't working for her, such as her cravings for candy at night. In short, Sarah had made progress. She had learned from her past attempts at dieting and exercising and was trying to continue some of the changes she'd made before, but she wasn't seeing her improvements. Why?

There are probably several reasons. For example, Sarah was fired from her job because she was having difficulty managing her workload and office relationships, in large part due to symptoms related to her bipolar disorder, such as depression, reduced motivation, difficulty concentrating, lack of interest, and irritability. Between her bipolar diagnosis and being fired, Sarah was more likely to see herself as a failure or think she wouldn't be able to manage her depression and effectively lose weight. These types of overly negative thoughts are common in people with bipolar disorder. In chapter 4, I'll describe cognitive restructuring, a skill that can help you change such thoughts.

A second reason that Sarah may not be seeing the positive changes she's made in her diet and exercise habits is that she has a very narrow definition of success, measuring it entirely by her weight. Therefore, she wasn't seeing the other changes she'd made in her life; she was just focused on one thing—that she had gained weight. This is a common pitfall for everyone, regardless of whether they have bipolar disorder. But as mentioned above, people with bipolar disorder are more likely to have more intense and more frequent negative thoughts than others. For this reason, it's likely that people with bipolar disorder will have a very narrow definition of success, leading to more intense negative thoughts if they don't meet that definition.

The Benefits of Setting Goals

Sarah's story highlights the pitfalls of not setting realistic goals and not acknowledging every bit of progress. Doing so can make you think you've failed when you're actually making progress and successfully engaging in small changes that make a difference in creating a healthier lifestyle. Clearly, whether you set achievable, appropriate goals can make or break your commitment to changing your diet, exercise patterns, and other lifestyle habits.

To give you an idea of how to set appropriate goals for creating a healthier lifestyle, let's consider another example.

Fred, who's in his midtwenties, was recently diagnosed with bipolar disorder. He currently lives at home with his mother and sister and takes classes part-time at a local college. Fred doesn't like to cook and therefore either eats the meals his mother cooks or buys his meals and snacks at coffee shops and restaurants. Fred also enjoys drinking beer in the evenings to "unwind," and although he tends to walk to class, he currently doesn't do any other forms of exercise.

What kinds of goals might Fred set to create a healthier lifestyle? The sample worksheet that follows shows some possibilities—all based on approaches presented later in this book.

Fred's Goal-Setting Worksheet

Identify three main goals for adopting a healthier lifestyle. Then identify how you'll accomplish those goals. What intermediate steps are necessary to achieve your main goals?

Main goal 1: *Lose weight. I want to lose 10 percent of my current weight, which would be thirty pounds.*

> **Intermediate goal 1:** *Record the foods I eat by using a daily food diary three days per week.*

> **Intermediate goal 2:** *Identify five healthy menu options at my favorite restaurants.*

> **Intermediate goal 3:** *Include my mom in my efforts to change my diet. Maybe I could have her read this book and ask her to make healthier substitutions in some of the meals she cooks.*

Main goal 2: *Increase my weekly physical activity by exercising three to four days per week for at least thirty minutes, at moderate intensity.*

> **Intermediate goal 1:** *Continue to walk to my classes.*

> **Intermediate goal 2:** *Start doing a new activity, like playing tennis or riding a bike.*

> **Intermediate goal 3:** *Ask my friends Sue and John to do something active together, like walking or going for a bike ride.*

Main goal 3: *Drink less alcohol—ultimately just three beers per week.*

> **Intermediate goal 1:** *Monitor my cravings so that I understand why they come up and how strong they are.*

> **Intermediate goal 2:** *Identify ways to unwind other than drinking beer, such as reading a book, watching a movie, or talking to a friend.*

> **Intermediate goal 3:** *Schedule evening activities that don't involve drinking.*

The Importance of Setting Realistic and Specific Goals

As you can see in the sample worksheet, Fred set very specific and realistic goals. For example, he didn't just plan to lose weight; he specified that he wanted to lose 10 percent of his current weight, or thirty pounds. He may actually want to lose more weight in the long run, but a goal of losing 5 to 10 percent of your body weight is more realistic, especially when you're just beginning to make changes to your lifestyle. And while losing just 5 to 10 percent of your current weight may not sound like much, data from a diabetes prevention study showed that losing 7 percent of your body weight can significantly reduce the risk of developing diabetes (Diabetes Prevention Program Research Group 1999; Knowler et al. 2002).

Furthermore, Fred made specific and achievable plans to change his lifestyle to increase the likelihood that he would successfully lose weight. Importantly, he also sought support from friends and family members to help him with his three main goals. This is crucial, and I'll discuss it at length in chapter 10.

How to Assess Whether Goals Are Realistic

How realistic a goal is depends on you and your previous experience with making healthy lifestyle changes. It's very individual. A goal that's realistic for one person may not be realistic for another. For example, if you've never really enjoyed exercising before or don't have much experience with exercise, then it probably wouldn't be realistic to plan to exercise three or four times per week initially. Instead, it might be best to increase your day-to-day activities—things you're already doing. This could mean walking an extra lap around the grocery store while shopping, checking your mail more than once per day if doing so involves a stairway or walking to a mailbox, or even getting up from your couch more frequently throughout the day. Any increase in activity—simply moving your body—will help you burn calories and become more fit and healthy. (I'll discuss increasing day-to-day activities at length in chapter 5.)

Setting realistic goals can be difficult. When we really want something, we tend to make big plans and set grand goals. Weight loss is a prime example. Over the years, I've had many people come into my office wanting to lose lots of weight—often more than 20 percent of their current weight. This isn't a realistic goal, whether you have bipolar disorder or not. Even for people who once weighed much less than they currently do, losing more than 5 to 10 percent of their current weight would be incredibly challenging. It isn't impossible, and some people with bipolar disorder have been successful in losing this much weight, but it isn't a good starting goal.

If you have big plans, such as running a marathon, cutting your calorie intake in half (say, from 3,400 calories per day to 1,700 calories per day), or losing fifty pounds, you must first develop smaller-scale goals to increase the likelihood that you'll reach these big goals. This is especially true for people with bipolar disorder, who already have the additional challenge of managing their illness, along with the tendency to think more negatively than people without bipolar disorder. Therefore, it's especially important that you put yourself in a position to succeed by setting very realistic, achievable goals. This will go a long way toward increasing positive thoughts. So if your major goal is to run ten miles, begin with the goal of walking two miles, then build up to running two miles, and so on.

Let's consider another example of whether goals are realistic.

Ten years ago, Joan was fired from her job for being irritable with coworkers. She's currently on disability, in part due to her bipolar disorder, which makes it difficult for her to work well with others when she's irritable during periods of depression. Joan has felt very isolated and alone since she stopped working. When she met with me, she said that one of her goals was being more social, which she defined as returning to work and having parties.

Do you think Joan's goals are realistic? It may be hard to tell without knowing more about her, but can you perhaps identify some intermediate, smaller goals? For example, instead of planning to be around groups of people at work or at parties, Joan could practice interacting with one person or a small group of friends first. She might also benefit from practicing people skills and effective communication strategies first. (Given that social support is such an important part of having a healthy lifestyle, I'll discuss some of these communication strategies in chapter 10.)

To determine whether a goal is realistic or not, try it for one week and see if you have trouble accomplishing it. If so, the goal is too difficult. It would probably be best to modify the goal to make it a bit less challenging and therefore more realistic. If you continue to have trouble making progress toward your goals, you need to continue to modify them, get more support from friends or family, or both. A key point to remember is that a goal can never be too easy. So continue to make a goal less challenging (or more realistic!) until you have a good chance of achieving it. Once you do, you can move on and set a more challenging goal. Given how crucial it is to set and achieve goals, in chapter 7 I'll review the key principles of goal setting and also discuss the importance of rewarding yourself for your accomplishments. If you think this would be particularly helpful for you in accomplishing your goals, you may want to read chapter 7 next.

How to Assess Whether Goals Are Specific

A key guideline in setting goals that are specific is that you should be able to measure your achievement. This allows you to know whether you've actually accomplished a goal. Consider the following two goals:

Goal 1: To run greater distances.

Goal 2: To start running one mile this week; then, for the next two weeks, run one mile and walk one mile; then try running two miles.

Obviously, one of these goals (goal 2) is specific enough to measure and the other is not. Here's another example:

Goal: To have a healthier diet by eating more fruits and vegetables.

Is this goal specific enough? This goal does clarify how this person wants to change his diet (by eating more fruits and vegetables), but how could he know whether he's accomplished his goal of eating more fruits and vegetables? Would eating one piece of fruit three days a week be enough? First, he would have to have an idea of how many fruits and vegetables he's currently eating. Let's say he determines that some days he doesn't eat any fruits or vegetables at all. In that case, he might set this more specific goal:

Revised goal: To have a healthier diet by consuming one piece of fruit or one serving of vegetables each day.

Now anyone can determine whether this has person accomplished his goal because it can be measured. One reason being able to measure a goal is so important is that it allows you to know how to modify it if it's too challenging. Having clear, specific goals also allows you to know when you've achieved them so that you can reward yourself for accomplishing them or set new goals—or better yet, both! And along the way, you'll be able to assess your progress toward creating a healthier lifestyle.

There is a potential downside to having specific goals: you'll also know when you haven't accomplished them. Unfortunately, people with bipolar disorder often see this as failing due to the increased tendency to think negatively. In chapter 4, I'll discuss negative thoughts in detail and also explain how to change them. This skill will come in handy if you have trouble accomplishing your initial goals. But remember, having trouble completing your goals means that they aren't realistic and need to be modified to make them more achievable.

Another tip when making goals is to describe them to someone else. Ask others if they would know whether you've accomplished your goal. If another person wouldn't be able to tell exactly when you've accomplished a goal, it probably isn't specific enough.

Exercise: Setting Some Initial Goals

Now it's time for you to start selecting some initial goals. You'll find a blank worksheet for this purpose here. A downloadable version of this worksheet is available at http://www.newharbinger.com/31304 (see the back of the book for instructions on how to access it). The downloadable version will come in handy as you continue to set new goals in the weeks and months to come.

As you fill out the worksheet, remember to choose goals that are realistic and specific. Of course, you may have more than three goals related to creating a healthier lifestyle, but I encourage you to just focus on three for now, as it can be difficult to make more than a few changes at one time. You can always add new goals later.

Goal-Setting Worksheet

Identify three main goals for adopting a healthier lifestyle. Then identify how you'll accomplish those goals. What intermediate steps are necessary to achieve your main goals?

Main goal 1: _____

    Intermediate goal 1: _____

    _____

    Intermediate goal 2: _____

    _____

    Intermediate goal 3: _____

    _____

Main goal 2: _____

    Intermediate goal 1: _____

    _____

    Intermediate goal 2: _____

    _____

    Intermediate goal 3: _____

    _____

Main goal 3: _____

    Intermediate goal 1: _____

    _____

    Intermediate goal 2: _____

    _____

    Intermediate goal 3: _____

    _____

Giving Yourself Homework

Now that you've established some goals, along with the intermediate steps necessary to achieve them, you should have some specific things to work on and practice. Therapists often call this practice "homework." The idea is to try making changes to your lifestyle when you aren't reading this book or gathering more information about a healthy lifestyle. It's vital for you to be an active participant in the process of changing your lifestyle. Just remember, by "being active," I don't mean committing yourself to making big changes all at once. In fact, I would caution you against doing this. Rather, the idea is to commit yourself to making realistic changes and to have concrete plans for doing so, taking it one small step at a time.

If you have trouble getting started or following through on your goals, revisit the exercise "Doing a Behavior Analysis" in chapter 1 and complete it again to help you move yourself out of the contemplation stage and into preparation and action. If you encounter obstacles to doing your homework, a behavior analysis will help you clarify the problem, which, in turn, will help you use this book to overcome the specific obstacles that stand in the way of achieving your goals.

Summary

- Setting goals is important to creating a healthy lifestyle.

- Goals should be both realistic and specific.

- A realistic goal is one that you can accomplish.

- A specific goal is one that you can measure.

- Realistic and specific goals are particularly important for people with bipolar disorder, who have a tendency to think that they're failing or to have many negative thoughts.

- The Goal-Setting Worksheet will help you structure your goals and the steps necessary to achieve them.

Chapter 3

Understanding Good Nutrition and a Balanced Diet

Chapter 2 addressed the importance of setting specific and realistic goals. Having clear goals will be essential as you read through this chapter on nutrition and begin to think about the kinds of changes you want to make to your diet. As discussed in chapter 1, your physical health can impact your bipolar disorder, and being in good physical health may increase the likelihood that you'll experience fewer bipolar symptoms or that your symptoms will be less intense. One key way to improve your physical health is to eat healthy, nutritious foods. Therefore, in this chapter I'll help you learn to identify which foods are best for you.

Over the years, there have been many popular diets that suggested focusing on eating or not eating certain foods or food groups. For example, some diets call for eating fewer carbohydrates and more protein. Other diets advocate cleansing the body by eating only fruits and vegetables. The approach I advocate is largely informed by recommendations of the Harvard School of Public Health, which are based on extensive research by experts in the field of nutrition (for example, Willett 2011). In brief, this approach encourages eating a balanced diet that includes a wide range of foods from the four major food groups—fruits, vegetables, healthy proteins, and whole grains—along with plenty of water.

If you think this sounds like fairly basic nutritional advice, you're correct. I stick to the basics of nutrition for two reasons. First, healthy eating relies on these basic principles of nutrition. And second, I'm not an expert on nutrition, so it would be beyond my training and expertise to offer in-depth advice on the subject. Fortunately, I've found that most people have a pretty good idea of which foods are healthy versus unhealthy, so I see my job as helping people make the choice to eat healthier foods. This is particularly important for people with bipolar disorder, who are often more likely to choose unhealthy foods due to mood swings and the effects of medications.

Just to be clear, in this book my focus is on making healthy choices. In this chapter, I'll review key principles of nutrition and also discuss some recent research on nutrients that may be particularly helpful for people with bipolar disorder (Sylvia, Peters, et al. 2013). Then, chapter 4 is dedicated to helping you make good choices about food. If you think you may have specific nutritional needs or dietary requirements, or if you think it would be helpful to have someone plan your meals, I encourage you to work with a dietitian or speak with your doctor.

Calories

In this nutritional overview, we'll look at the basics, starting with calories. A *calorie* is a measure of food energy. Technically speaking, 1 calorie is the amount of energy needed to raise the temperature of 1 gram of water by 1 degree Celsius. More simply put, the calories in food provide energy—the same energy you'd need to burn to lose weight. Thus, the more energy you eat by consuming calories, the more exercise or activity you need to do to burn this energy; otherwise it will be stored by your body, often as fat. For this reason, knowing the number of calories you eat each day can be a useful strategy in losing weight.

The amount of calories a person needs daily depends on many factors, including activity level, gender, age, and weight. But for most people who aren't very active, average daily calorie consumption shouldn't exceed about 2,000 calories.

And while it's important to monitor your daily calorie intake, be aware that simply knowing the number of calories in a serving of food isn't enough. You also need to consider how nutritious a food is, in terms of vitamin and mineral content. For example, 200 calories from cheese puffs or a candy bar won't provide the same nutritional benefit as 200 calories from a green salad, fresh fruit, or whole grain bread. That said, be aware that some foods that are highly nutritious may also be high in calories. For example, almonds can be a nutritious part of a balanced diet, but because they're very high in calories, with just ¼ cup having 207 calories, they should be consumed in moderation.

Calories can also sneak up in beverages, which people tend to overlook as part of their diet. Consider these examples:

- 12 ounces of soda: up to 190 calories

- 12 ounces of bottled sweetened water: up to 140 calories

- 5 ounces of wine: about 120 calories

- 12 ounces of beer: typically about 150 calories

- 8 ounces of orange juice: over 100 calories

- 8 ounces of apple juice: up to 120 calories

- 8 ounces of whole milk: over 140 calories

- 8 ounces of skim milk: about 80 calories

- 8 ounces of nondairy milk: as much as 120 calories

As you can see, these calories can really add up. Yet because beverages aren't as filling as food, you're likely to eat a similar amount of food whether or not you drink calorie-dense beverages. This is one of the many reasons why water is such an excellent beverage—a topic I'll revisit in depth later in the chapter.

The Building Blocks of Foods

The nutrients in foods can be divided into two categories: *macronutrients* and *micronutrients*. The primary macronutrients are carbohydrates, proteins, and fats. Micronutrients include vitamins and minerals, along with some of the building blocks of proteins and fats. For the most part, I won't be getting into the details of micronutrients, but it's helpful to understand the distinction. (And don't worry: you haven't accidentally picked up a textbook on nutrition! I just need to make sure you understand a few basics of nutrition before we start looking at healthy dietary choices.)

Carbohydrates

Carbohydrates are a major component of most foods from plant sources: fruits, vegetables, grains, beans, nuts, and seeds. They can be divided into two main groups: *simple carbohydrates* (sugars) and *complex carbohydrates* (what many people think of as starches).

A subcategory of complex carbohydrates is *fiber*. Having sufficient fiber in your diet is important for health. It's also great for weight loss, because it's mostly indigestible, so it doesn't contribute calories, but it helps you feel full. It also helps slow the release of sugars into the bloodstream, so it reduces risk of diabetes. When you consume complex carbohydrates other than fiber, your body breaks them down into their component sugars. Each gram of carbohydrate, whether complex or simple, has about 4 calories.

Although carbohydrates often get a bad rap, be aware that your body is designed to use them for energy, so they're an important part of the diet. Many of the ill effects of carbohydrates stem from excessive consumption of sugars and refined carbohydrates (a topic I'll address later), so keep your focus on consuming complex carbohydrates in whole grains, vegetables, fruits, and beans.

Proteins

Proteins are found in many foods. They're most abundant in meat, poultry, seafood, and eggs, but they're also present in many other foods, especially beans and peas. The building blocks of proteins are amino acids. When you eat proteins, your body breaks them down into their component amino acids. What distinguishes one protein from another is which amino acids are present and the order in which they're arranged. In terms of dietary sources, proteins from animal sources are *complete proteins*, meaning they contain all of the amino acids you need to consume in your diet. Those from plant sources generally aren't complete, but if you consume a wide variety of plant foods, you'll probably get all of the individual amino acids your body needs. Each gram of protein has about 4 calories.

Proteins are, of course, an important component of the diet for maintaining muscle. However, they also play many other essential roles in the body, including in *neurotransmitters*—chemicals that transmit messages in the brain. Because many sources of protein are also high in fat (like bacon) or salt (such as processed meats), it's best to keep your focus on healthy choices such as lean meats, seafood, poultry, and legumes.

Fats

Like proteins, fats are found in many foods, but in terms of diet, they're most abundant in meat, dairy products, nuts, seeds, and cooking oils. There are two main types of fats: *saturated fats* and *unsaturated fats*. Saturated fats, which tend to be solid at room temperature, are found in high amounts in cheese, butter, and meats, as well as coconut oil.

Unsaturated fats, which are often liquid at room temperature, are present in foods such as avocados, nuts, canola oil, olive oil, and other vegetable oils. Each gram of fat has about 9 calories, which is more than twice as many calories per gram as carbohydrates or proteins.

Fats do play a role in helping our bodies function. For example, they are a key component of cell membranes, and they're necessary for healthy skin. In the brain, they form sheaths around neurons that enable them to function and help them carry messages more quickly. They're also needed for the body to absorb certain vitamins and to make hormones. So don't try to avoid fat altogether. Instead, opt for a moderate intake of healthy fats—primarily unsaturated fats, and especially omega-3 fatty acids (which I'll discuss later in this chapter).

Also, be aware that some evidence suggests that reducing intake of saturated fats can help reduce the risk of cardiovascular disease (Hooper et al. 2011). As discussed in chapter 1, this is particularly crucial for people with bipolar disorder, who might be at greater risk for developing cardiovascular disease than people without bipolar disorder.

The Fundamentals of a Healthy Diet

Now that we've covered those fundamental facts about nutrition, we can take a look at what you're probably interested in: how to make healthy choices about what to eat and how much to eat. For this discussion, I'll mainly draw upon the current recommendations on healthy eating from the US Department of Agriculture (USDA), which are summarized in the MyPlate diagram that follows.

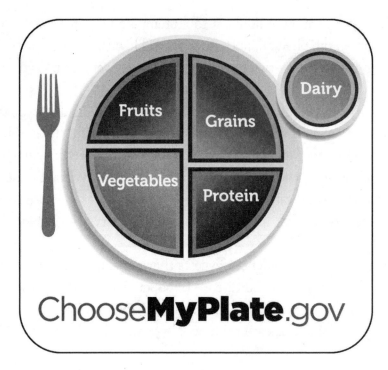

US Department of Agriculture

These guidelines were developed by the USDA's Center for Nutrition Policy and Promotion, which was established in 1994 to improve the nutrition and well-being of the US population. All foods are allowed as part of this diet; it doesn't dictate that there are forbidden foods that shouldn't be eaten. Instead, the goal is to eat healthy amounts of foods from the major food groups—fruits, vegetables, healthy proteins, whole grains, and possibly dairy—while minimizing consumption of foods that have little or no nutritional value (candy, chips, soda, and so on). The figure gives a rough idea of the relative amount of each food group you should eat at each meal (or over the course of each day, if that works better for you). In the sections that follow, I'll give more details on each food group. For a wealth of detailed information, including recommendations tailored specifically to your age, gender, and activity level, visit http://www.choosemyplate.gov.

Fruits

Fruits are generally a healthy choice. Most fruits are low in calories and fat while also being a great source of fiber and certain vitamins and minerals, especially vitamin C and potassium. If you turn to the table "Nutrients in Select Foods," a bit later in this chapter, you'll see that some fruits, such as bananas and pears, are very high in carbohydrates, which the body converts into sugars during digestion. Therefore, it may be wise to consume fruits that are lower in carbohydrates. However, given that fruits contain valuable vitamins and minerals, I usually suggest that people not worry about the amount of sugar in fruit. You can cut sugar from your diet in other places, such as eating fewer desserts. Fruit is also a more healthy choice than most snacks people tend to eat. However, the high sugar content in fruit can be an issue with fruit juices, where you're getting all of the sugar without the fiber that helps slow the release of those sugars into the bloodstream. So try to eat fruit "naked," in its whole form, as much as possible, rather than in processed forms such as jams, pies, and juices, which are typically high in sugar.

The USDA (2014) suggests that most people eat 1½ to 2 cups of fruit per day. (For more complete details on what counts as 1 cup, visit http://www.choosemyplate.gov/food -groups/fruits-counts.html). Or you can just use the MyPlate diagram for guidance, making fruit a little less than one-quarter of your plate at each meal.

Vegetables

Vegetables are very healthy. On their own, they're generally low in fat and calories and a great source of fiber, vitamins, and minerals. And because they're so diverse, everyone should be able to find vegetables they enjoy eating. That said, different vegetables contain different nutrients. The best way to get well-rounded nutrition is to eat a rainbow of vegetables, from dark leafy greens to ripe red peppers. Unfortunately, one of the most popular vegetables—potatoes—also tends to be less nutritious, so try to opt for other vegetables whenever you can.

The USDA (2014) suggests that most people eat from 2½ to 3 cups of vegetables per day. (For more complete details on what counts as 1 cup, visit http://www.choosemyplate .gov/food-groups/vegetables-amount.html). Or you can just use the MyPlate diagram for guidance, making vegetables a little more than one-quarter of your plate at each meal.

Healthy Proteins

Protein is an essential part of your diet, but it's important to choose healthy proteins. The USDA's MyPlate recommendations include meat, poultry, seafood, beans, peas, eggs, soy products, nuts, and seeds in this group. The USDA recommends at least 8 ounces of cooked seafood per week, and also specifies that meat and poultry choices should be lean or low-fat. For an example of why this is important, take a look at the table "Nutrients in Select Foods." In the section on proteins, you can see that 3 ounces of ground beef with 30 percent fat contains 25 grams of fat, whereas the same amount of lean ground beef, with just 10 percent fat, contains only 9 grams of fat. Good choices include fish and the white meat of chicken without skin (the dark meat and skin are higher in fat).

The USDA (2014) suggests that most people eat 5 to 6 "ounce equivalents" of foods that are high-quality sources of protein daily. (For more complete details on what counts as an ounce equivalent, visit http://www.choosemyplate.gov/food-groups/protein-foods -counts.html). Or you can just use the MyPlate diagram for guidance, making protein about one-quarter of your plate at each meal.

Whole Grains

Grains are an important source of carbohydrates; however, some grains can be considered *empty calories*—calories from foods that contain little nutritional value other than the calories. You can easily distinguish grain-based foods that are nutritious from those that aren't by identifying whether they contain whole or refined grains. *Whole grains* contain all of the parts of the grain: the germ, endosperm, and bran. *Refined grains* contain only the endosperm; examples include white flour or white rice. When buying packaged foods, consult the ingredients section of the label, which will list whole grains as such. Keep an eye out for the word "whole" to ensure that you're consuming mostly whole grains.

The USDA (2014) suggests that most people eat 5 to 6 "ounce equivalents" of grains daily, and that at least half that amount be in the form of whole grains. (For more complete details on what counts as an ounce equivalent, visit http://www.choosemyplate.gov /food-groups/grains.html). Or you can just use the MyPlate diagram for guidance, making whole grains about one-quarter of your plate at each meal.

Nutrients in Select Foods

Food	Calories	Protein (g)	Carbs (g)	Fat (g)
Fruits				
Apple with skin (raw, medium)	81	<1	21	<1
Banana (raw, medium)	105	1	27	1
Blackberries (raw, 1 cup)	74	1	18	1
Blueberries (raw, 1 cup)	82	1	21	1
Cantaloupe (raw, 1 cup)	57	1	13	<1
Cherries (raw, 10 medium)	49	1	11	1
Grapefruit (raw, ½ medium)	37	1	10	<1
Grapes (raw, ½ cup)	29	<1	8	<1
Melon (raw, 1 cup)	66	2	15	1
Nectarine (raw, medium)	67	1	16	1
Orange (raw, medium)	65	1	16	<1
Peach (raw, medium)	37	1	10	<1
Pear (raw, medium)	98	1	25	1
Pineapple (raw, ½ cup)	38	<1	10	<1
Raspberries (raw, 1 cup)	61	1	14	1
Strawberries (raw, 1 cup)	45	1	11	1
Watermelon (raw, 1 cup)	50	1	12	1
Vegetables				
Asparagus (boiled, ½ cup)	22	2	4	<1
Broccoli (boiled, ½ cup)	23	2	4	<1
Carrots (boiled, ½ cup)	35	1	8	<1
Celery (raw, ½ cup)	11	<1	3	<1
Corn (boiled, ½ cup)	89	3	21	1
Cucumber (raw, ½ cup)	7	<1	2	<1
Eggplant (raw, ½ cup)	11	1	3	<1
Green beans (boiled, ½ cup)	22	1	5	<1
Peas (boiled, ½ cup)	67	5	13	<1
Potato (scalloped, ½ cup)	105	4	13	5

Food	Calories	Protein (g)	Carbs (g)	Fat (g)
Proteins				
Beef, ground (30% fat, 3 oz)	279	12	<1	25
Beef, ground (10% fat, 3 oz)	182	23	<1	9
Cashews (1 oz)	165	5	9	14
Chicken, breast, skinless (3 oz)	140	27	<1	3
Egg, boiled (1 large)	77	6	1	5
Lamb, chop (lean, 3 oz)	150	17	<1	6
Haddock, baked (3 oz)	95	21	<1	1
Peanuts (shelled, 1 oz)	166	7	5	14
Pork, chop (lean, 3 oz)	185	24	<1	9
Salmon, baked (3 oz)	175	60	<1	25
Swordfish, baked (3 oz)	132	22	<1	4
Turkey, ground (7% fat, 4 oz)	128	16	<1	7
Turkey, ground (15% fat, 4 oz)	153	14	<1	11
Grains				
Bread, wheat (1 slice)	61	2	11	1
Bread, white (1 slice)	64	2	12	1
English muffin, whole wheat (½)	68	2	13	1
Bagel, whole wheat (½)	82	3	16	1
Cereal, Cheerios (1 oz)	111	1	20	2
Cereal, cornflakes (1 oz)	110	2	25	1
Pancakes (4 inches in diameter, 1)	62	2	9	2
Pasta, enriched, cooked (½ cup)	100	3	19	1
Rice, enriched, cooked (½ cup)	141	4	50	<1
Rice, long-grain brown (1 cup)	216	5	50	1
Rice, long-grain white (1 cup)	223	4	50	<1

Dairy

The USDA's MyPlate recommendations include consuming some dairy each day, largely because milk is a primary source of three important nutrients: calcium, potassium, and vitamin D (which is added to fortified milk). Thus, dairy products may help with bone health (Rice, Quann, and Miller 2013). However, there are many other sources of calcium, potassium, and vitamin D, so dairy may not be a necessary component of a healthy diet. Plus, dairy products can be relatively high in calories, which is why the MyPlate recommendations specify fat-free or low-fat dairy products. Note that milk is especially high in calories for a beverage. For example, 8 ounces (1 cup) of 2% milk has 122 calories, so drinking three 8-ounce servings per day would add 366 calories to your diet. So you might consider instead drinking water—a no-calorie beverage that's essential for health. In short, dairy need not be an essential part of your diet, as long as you get calcium, potassium, and vitamin D from other sources.

Water

Water, and lots of it, is an absolutely vital component of a healthy diet (Popkin, D'Anci, and Rosenberg 2010). Here are some good reasons to make water a big part of your daily diet:

- **Water helps maintain the balance of body fluids.** Your body is composed of about 60 percent water, and bodily fluids play a key role in digestion, absorption, circulation, transportation of nutrients, and maintaining body temperature.

- **Water has no calories.** When you're thirsty, you need to drink something, but many beverages are laden with either calories or artificial sweeteners. Not water! It's a healthy substitution for higher-calorie beverages and therefore can be useful for controlling your daily calorie intake.

- **Water can energize muscles.** If your body doesn't have adequate water, your muscles may not work as well, leading to muscle fatigue and poor athletic performance. Therefore, the American College of Sports Medicine (2005) recommends that people drink about 17 ounces of water (a little over 2 cups) approximately two hours before exercise. They also recommend that, during exercise, people start drinking water early and continue to drink at regular intervals to replace fluids lost by sweating.

- **Water may keep skin looking good.** Your skin needs water to stay healthy. If you're dehydrated or aren't drinking enough water, your skin will probably look more dry and wrinkled.

- **Water helps you think.** You also need water for proper functioning of your brain, including to help you concentrate, stay alert, and remember things. In addition, dehydration can cause headaches.

The amount of water you need depends on your gender, age, and weight. It also depends on your diet, as some foods, such as many fruits, have a very high water content. Approximately 20 percent of your water probably comes from food, but the other 80 percent comes from what you drink. According to the Institute of Medicine (2014), men need about 4 quarts of water per day, or sixteen 8-ounce glasses (in addition to food), and women need about 3 quarts per day, or eleven 8-ounce glasses. Again, if you're well hydrated, you'll usually urinate several times per day, and your urine will be pale yellow.

Nutrition for Bipolar Disorder

Recent research suggests that specific nutrients may be beneficial for the brain and help it function well. This is a key consideration for people with bipolar disorder because it's a disease of the brain, caused (at least in part) by abnormal functioning of brain cells.

Researchers have begun to find evidence suggesting that certain nutrients may be particularly helpful for alleviating bipolar disorder. For example, omega-3 fatty acids, a type of polyunsaturated fat, are believed to calm communication between neurons in a way that eases depression (Balanzá-Martínez et al. 2011). Many types of fish are high in omega-3 fatty acids, which is one reason why seafood is considered a very healthy food choice. Omega-3 fatty acids can also be taken as a supplement. Given that omega-3 fatty acids are one of the best-studied nutritional supplements, it seems safe to recommend them for people who have bipolar disorder. However, it's always best to consult with your doctor before making major changes in your diet or taking a new supplement. That said, it can almost never hurt to eat more fish.

Folate (or folic acid, a B vitamin) is another micronutrient that may improve depression. It can help elevate levels of serotonin, a neurotransmitter that seems to be in short supply in people who are depressed (Mischoulon and Raab 2007). Good sources of folate include dark green leafy vegetables, fruits, nuts, beans, peas, dairy products, chicken, beef, eggs, and seafood. Spinach, liver, yeast, asparagus, and Brussels sprouts are among the foods with the highest levels of folate. The nutrient magnesium, found in leafy greens, avocadoes, and bananas, may help reduce agitation—which is similar to some symptoms of mania—as folate helps reduce depression (Sylvia, Peters, et al. 2013).

Be aware that you may need to take a supplement in order to get the benefits from any of these nutrients. This will ensure that you get a large enough dose to be helpful. Unfortunately, data on how much of each nutrient to take and its exact benefits is still unclear, especially regarding bipolar disorder. Therefore, I usually encourage people to just follow the key nutritional principles described above, eating a balanced diet as shown in the MyPlate figure. This is often sufficient to ensure that you're getting the right amount of micronutrients, or at least that you aren't deficient in any nutrients. If you think a more specific dietary plan may be helpful for you, I encourage you to talk to a dietitian or other health professional who can help you create a plan tailored specifically to you.

Overweight and Obesity

You are probably aware that more and more people are becoming overweight, especially in the United States. And I'm sure I don't need to explain the health consequences of being overweight. These are widely known. Yet people in general, and especially people with bipolar disorder, continue to struggle with maintaining a healthy weight. If this applies to you, as it does to many of my clients, the rest of this chapter and chapter 4 will help you start turning the situation around.

The first question is, how can you tell if you're overweight or obese? The most common measure is something called the body mass index (BMI), a measurement obtained by dividing weight by height in inches squared, then multiplying by 703. Fortunately, it isn't necessary to do the math. You can find many BMI calculators online. (I often use one you can find at http://www.cdc.gov/healthyweight/assessing/bmi.) A BMI between 25 and 30 is considered overweight, and a BMI over 30 is considered obese.

Either condition is a significant health concern, but obesity is more extreme, with excess body fat accumulating to the extent that it can lead to reduced life expectancy (Haslam and James 2005). If you're obese, this is a serious issue and you need to discuss it with your doctor.

However, in working with people with bipolar disorder, I've found that focusing on BMI and labels such as "obese" may not be especially helpful in losing weight and adopting a healthier lifestyle. As discussed in previous chapters, having bipolar disorder means that you're more likely to judge yourself, and especially to judge yourself negatively. For this reason, I typically encourage people with bipolar disorder to not get overly focused on losing weight when making healthy lifestyle choices. There are many ways to improve your lifestyle other than losing weight, such as becoming more physically active, eating a more nutritious diet, reducing substance use, or making changes to improve your sleep. Yet losing excess weight has enormous health benefits, such as reducing your risk of heart disease and even cancer (Wing et al. 2011), so it is worth doing.

And given that we're focusing on diet in both this chapter and the next, I'll go ahead and give you the secret to losing weight: burn more calories than you eat. If you do this, you will lose weight. Burning more calories than you eat requires that you do two things: don't eat too many calories, and exercise more often or more strenuously to burn more calories. These two steps may be particularly difficult if you have bipolar disorder because depression can increase cravings for high-calorie comfort foods while also sapping your energy and motivation to exercise. Therefore, in the rest of this chapter and chapter 4, I'll offer many tips that will help you choose foods with fewer calories. Then, in chapters 5 and 6, I'll provide strategies that can help you get more physical activity. The good news is, if you follow these recommendations, you can lose weight—despite having bipolar disorder, experiencing depression, and taking medications that sometimes lead to weight gain.

Diet Makeover

Now that you're aware that calories and saturated fats can contribute to obesity and poor health, let's discuss how you can make changes to your diet to reduce your intake of calories and unhealthy fats. There are many recipes available online and in cooking magazines that can help you make meals that are low in calories and fat, and scores of cookbooks are devoted to this topic—but what about making changes to what you're already eating?

Below, I've provided an example of how you can reduce calories and fat by making slightly different choices. The two columns on the left show a sample diet and the number of calories in each food. The middle column, "Nutritional change," offers suggestions on how to modify each meal to reduce the amount of calories consumed and bring the diet more in line with the USDA's MyPlate recommendations. Finally, the two right-hand columns provide specific substitutions that fulfill the recommendations in the middle column and the number of calories in these new, more nutritious choices.

Sample Diet Makeover

Original Meal Plan	Calories	Nutritional changes	Revised, Healthier Meal Plan	Calories
Breakfast				
Plain bagel with 2 tbsp of honey-walnut cream cheese	350	Choose foods with less fat and calories.	Whole grain cereal with ½ cup skim milk	173
Milk, 2%, 1 cup	130	Use low-fat or skim milk.	Milk, skim, 1 cup	90
Coffee, 1 cup, with 2 tbsp half-and-half	61		Coffee, 1 cup, with 2 tbsp skim milk	14
Total calories	541		Total calories	277
Snack				
Potato chips (1 oz)	160	Choose a lower fat alternative.	Grapes (1 oz)	30
Total calories	160		Total calories	30
Lunch				
2 slices of wheat bread with 1 tbsp mayonnaise	240	Choose foods with less fat, including lean meat.	2 slices of wheat bread with 1 tbsp hummus	180
Salami, 1 oz	71		Turkey breast, 1 oz	30
Cheddar cheese, 2 oz	226		½ Roma tomato	10
Doritos (1 oz)	150	Limit portion sizes.	Reduced-fat cheddar cheese, 1 oz	70
			Celery sticks, ½ cup	10
Total calories	687		Total calories	300

Dinner				
Chicken, fried, 3 oz	250	Use different cooking methods.	Lemon pepper chicken, baked, 3 oz	140
French fries, 2.5 oz	231		Hash browns, ½ cup	70
Asparagus, sautéed, ½ cup	153	Use lower-fat options.	Asparagus, boiled, with garlic salt, ½ cup	25
Ketchup, 1 tbsp	19	Limit consumption of sweets.	Ketchup, 1 tbsp	19
House salad with 2 tbsp ranch dressing	280		House salad with 2 tbsp fat-free ranch dressing	180
Brownie, chocolate fudge, 2-inch square	240		1 orange	69
Total calories	1,173		Total calories	503

Total calories for the day originally: 2,561

Total calories for the day with the makeover: 1,110

Total calories saved: 1,451

Many of the changes in the sample diet makeover involve selecting lower-fat foods, such as substituting 2% milk for skim milk or limiting portion size. Others are achieved by cooking foods differently or making completely different food choices, such as eating an orange for dessert rather than a brownie. Amazingly, by making these changes, you can save 1,451 calories—almost as much as the total recommended daily intake of calories for most people (approximately 2,000 calories).

Keeping Track of Your Nutrition: Food Labels

In 1990, the Congress passed the Nutrition Labeling and Education Act, which gave the Food and Drug Administration the authority to require nutritional labels on most packaged foods. These Nutrition Facts labels list both the nutritional content and number of calories per serving of the food, making it much easier for people to both improve their nutrition and lose weight. It's worthwhile to get familiar with these labels, so take a look at the example I've provided here.

Nutrition Facts

Serving Size 2/3 cup (55g)
Servings Per Container About 8

Amount Per Serving

Calories 230   Calories from Fat 72

	% Daily Value*
Total Fat 8g	**12%**
Saturated Fat 1g	**5%**
Trans Fat 0g	
Cholesterol 0mg	**0%**
Sodium 160mg	**7%**
Total Carbohydrate 37g	**12%**
Dietary Fiber 4g	**16%**
Sugars 1g	
Protein 3g	
Vitamin A	10%
Vitamin C	8%
Calcium	20%
Iron	45%

* Percent Daily Values are based on a 2,000 calorie diet. Your daily value may be higher or lower depending on your calorie needs.

	Calories:	2,000	2,500
Total Fat	Less than	65g	80g
Sat Fat	Less than	20g	25g
Cholesterol	Less than	300mg	300mg
Sodium	Less than	2,400mg	2,400mg
Total Carbohydrate		300g	375g
Dietary Fiber		25g	30g

US Food and Drug Administration

A key aspect of Nutrition Facts labels is that, at the very top, they provide information for a *specific serving size*. This is very important! A can of peanuts or a bag of chips may contain several servings, so you probably shouldn't eat the whole thing in one sitting. If you do, you need to multiply the nutritional and calorie content on the Nutrition Facts label by the "servings per container" number. In short, don't assume that the information on the Nutrition Facts label refers to the entire amount of food in the package. Food labels can also be tricky because the "% Daily Value" information assumes that you're eating 2,000 calories per day. Therefore, these percentages may be an underestimate if you're trying to eat under 2,000 calories, or an overestimate if you're consuming 2,500 calories or more per day, as so many people do.

Despite these potentially confusing aspects of Nutrition Facts labels, they are very helpful in tracking your calories and nutritional intake. In chapter 4, I'll take that process one step further and explain how to keep a food diary so that you can become an expert on your diet. That way you'll know exactly what changes you need to make to eat foods that are healthier and, if you're trying to lose weight, less calorie dense.

Summary

- Eating a more nutritious diet can improve your mental and physical health.

- Good nutrition means having a balanced diet.

- A balanced diet consists of fruits, vegetables, whole grains, and healthy proteins in the amounts shown on the USDA's MyPlate diagram.

- Drinking a lot of water is good for your health.

- Certain nutrients may be helpful for managing bipolar disorder, but experiencing these benefits typically requires taking supplements, rather than just making changes to your diet.

- Monitoring how many calories and how much fat you consume each day may help you lose weight.

- Food labels can be very helpful in tracking your daily calorie intake and assessing the nutritional value of the foods you eat.

Chapter 4

Changing Your Diet

There are typically two issues that people have with their diet. First, as discussed in chapter 3, people have difficulty eating nutritiously, in a way that's in keeping with the USDA's MyPlate recommendations. Second, people simply tend to eat too much. In this chapter, I'll provide guidance on how you can eat more nutritiously and consume smaller portion sizes. Many of these tips are especially geared toward people with bipolar disorder because they address how to manage negative thoughts and feelings, which are often triggers for eating unhealthy foods or eating too much.

The Importance of Monitoring Your Diet

The first step to changing your diet is to monitor what you eat. Tracking your daily intake of foods and beverages is an important tool if you are to control your diet. It will help you do all of the following:

- Understand your eating patterns

- Identify your dietary trouble spots

- Set goals

- Modify your goals

- Clarify why you do or do not lose weight

- Understand how nutritious your diet is

Let me give you an example to help you understand some of these reasons better. I love candy corns, those small, sugary, orange-and-yellow Halloween candies. Candy corns are loaded with high-fructose corn syrup and have no nutritional value. Therefore, candy corns can lead to weight gain if I consume more of the sugar in them than my body needs, which, beyond a certain point, will be stored as fat. As I'm writing this chapter, it's close to Halloween, and therefore I'm buying more of these candies because they're popular at this time of year. Once I open a bag, I tend to snack on them by grabbing a handful every time I walk by. When I'm not monitoring my diet, I don't pay attention to how many candy corns I'm eating, nor when I tend to eat them. Instead, I just notice when I've finished a bag of them and make a mental note that I need to buy more. What do you think would happen if I began to keep a record of every time I ate a few candy corns?

You might think, *Who cares? Having a few candy corns can't hurt anyone.* You'd be correct. Like almost any food, candy corns, if eaten in moderation, won't have harmful effects on the body. However, am I really eating just a few? It's impossible to answer this question if I don't write down how many candy corns I'm actually eating. If I were to start monitoring my daily food consumption, I'd also learn when I tend to snack on candy corns—for example, after a meal, while watching TV, or in the evenings—as well as the exact amount I'm eating. Only then can I set realistic goals for cutting down on my consumption of candy corns. For example, if I'm eating about thirty pieces, or four handfuls a day, I might begin by setting the goal of eating only twenty pieces this week. By monitoring my intake of candy and other foods in this way, I'll develop a better understanding of how my diet, in terms of both food choices and calorie consumption, contributes to my weight and overall nutrition.

How to Monitor Your Daily Food Consumption

There are many different ways to record what you eat, but the most basic is with written daily diaries. I've included an example a bit later in this chapter, as well as a blank form for your use. The first step is to write down all of the foods and beverages you consume each day and the amount of each.

It would be worthwhile to use a small, inexpensive digital kitchen scale, along with measuring cups, to accurately measure how much you're eating. After doing that for a while, you should be able to estimate amounts fairly easily. However, if you prefer to guess-timate, you can use the following Visual Guide to Serving Sizes.

Visual Guide to Serving Sizes

Standard serving size	Visual guide	Description
3 ounces of meat, poultry, or fish		A deck of cards the size of your palm
1 cup of vegetables; 1 cup of dry cereal		The size of your fist
1 medium piece of fruit		The size of a baseball
½ cup of cooked grains or pasta		A scoop of ice cream
1½ ounces of cheese		Four dice
1 teaspoon of oil		The tip of your thumb

Another important point is that you need to be specific and be sure to include each element of a meal. While it may be tempting to write something like "egg and cheese sandwich," this wouldn't be sufficiently accurate. Instead, each ingredient should have its own line: for example, 1 egg, 1 teaspoon of butter, 1 English muffin, and 1 ounce of cheese. Here's a sample food diary, completed by Ted, to give you an idea of how it should look.

Ted's Food Diary

Breakfast (amount and type of food or drink)	Calories
2 cups of orange juice	220
1 cup of black coffee	5
1 whole wheat English muffin	120
2 tbsp of chunky peanut butter	200
1 cup of water	0
Lunch (amount and type of food or drink)	Calories
2 slices of thin whole wheat bread	200
2 slices of turkey breast	120
2 slices of Swiss cheese	140
1 pickle	1
2 lettuce leaves	1
1 tbsp of mayonnaise (not low-fat)	90
1 tsp of mustard	3
8 oz of Diet Coke	1
1 oz of Sun Chips	140

Dinner (amount and type of food or drink)	Calories
2 oz hamburger (85% lean)	300
1 whole wheat hamburger bun	120
1 tsp ketchup	9
1 tsp mustard	3
2 cups of long-grain rice	432
1 tsp butter	36
2 cups of steamed broccoli	110
2 cups of Breyer's chocolate chip ice cream	568
2 cups of water	0
Snacks (amount and type of food or drink)	Calories
1.9 oz Snickers bar	250
2.4 oz chocolate chip Clif bar	230
4 cups of water	0
1 package of peanut butter and cracker sandwiches	140
Total calories for the day	3,439

Once you think that you've recorded everything you consumed over the course of the day, go back and try to determine how many calories each food or beverage has. As discussed in chapter 3, monitoring calories is important for managing your weight. The only way you can lose weight is to consume fewer calories than you burn through activity. Later in the book, I'll provide some guidelines on how to determine how many calories you're burning. Right now, let's consider how you can figure out how many calories you're eating.

This can be a time-consuming process, but there are some helpful tools. For example, if you enjoy using technology, there are phone apps and computer programs you can download that provide the number of calories in many common foods and beverages. So if you enter, for example, "1 Lender's onion bagel" into your online food diary, the number of calories in this food automatically pops up: 210 calories. One of my favorites programs is available at http://www.calorieking.com, but a web search on daily food diaries will give you many options.

Many of these online programs and applications offer the option of entering your own recipes for homemade foods. So after you've entered them once, you're set. And some of these programs allow you to track other health-related information, such as amount and type of exercise, amount of sleep, and even your daily mood. Although all of this information may be helpful, keep in mind the tip from chapter 2 about setting realistic goals: make small, step-by-step changes that you think you can maintain. So, although electronic wellness trackers can be handy, and perhaps exciting to use initially, they may require that you monitor too many different things at the outset, increasing the likelihood that you'll have difficulty sticking with the tracking. But don't despair! You can also keep a written food diary and use online resources or apps to determine the number of calories in various foods, including your own recipes.

The food diary doesn't track daily servings, serving sizes, or how well you're sticking to good nutritional recommendations. But as mentioned in chapter 3, at each meal, your plate will ideally be filled about halfway with fruits and vegetables, with whole grains and healthy proteins each occupying about one-fourth of your plate. This translates to consuming about one serving of each food group—fruits, vegetables, whole grains, and healthy proteins—per meal. This would be three servings of each food group per day. However, you can have more than three servings of whole grains and healthy proteins per day: six of whole grains and five of healthy proteins. You can also have more than three servings of nonstarchy vegetables, as long as they're not prepared with too much oil, butter, or other unhealthy or high-fat ingredients.

People often eat more than one serving of various food groups at a given meal. That's fine. As long as your plate at each meal—or your total food consumption over the course of the day—generally reflects the proportions in the MyPlate figure, chances are you're eating a nutritious diet. That said, be careful not to cram food onto your plate or choose a very big plate. For example, you could pile two 3-ounce hamburgers on whole wheat buns on one-quarter of your plate, but this would be all of your protein and most of your whole grains for the entire day. As for plate size, I recommend using smaller plates. I bet you'll find that you eat less food if you opt for a smaller plate. In short, it's important to pay attention to serving sizes.

Using the Information in Your Food Diary

Keeping a food diary will help you take control of your diet as you come to understand your consumption patterns and identify trouble spots in your diet. To see how this works, take a minute to review the sample food diary earlier in the chapter. How healthy does this diet seem? Keeping in mind the MyPlate figure and the basics of nutrition discussed in chapter 3, can you identify one or two things Ted is doing well? Would you suggest any changes or improvements?

Looking at Ted's food diary, you'll see that Ted made some excellent choices overall, such as eating whole grains, having several servings of vegetables, and not consuming too much of any food group. However, he could improve in several areas. For example, Ted had several unhealthy snacks, such as candy, peanut butter crackers, and chips. Ted could also benefit from choosing some lower-fat alternatives, such as low-fat peanut butter or low-fat ice cream and leaner meat to make his hamburger.

Importantly, the sample food diary also reveals that Ted consumed a lot of calories on this particular day: almost 3,500, which is about 1,500 calories more than recommended for the average man and about 1,800 more than recommended for the average woman. Unless Ted is extremely active, eating that many calories on a regular basis will lead to weight gain. Portion control could be very helpful here. By eating only 1 cup of rice at dinner and 1 cup of ice cream for dessert, Ted could save 500 calories.

Before we go on, I want to address an important point. As you read through the sample food diary, did you find yourself comparing it to your diet? Perhaps you thought that your diet is so much worse and felt as though you'll never be able to eat better. This kind of judgment is common among people in general, but it's much more likely for you, given that you have bipolar disorder. Remember, your brain tends to make more frequent and intense negative judgments. Please be kind to yourself as you try to change your lifestyle. This is hard work! Fortunately, there are effective strategies to help modify or replace negative thoughts, and I'll share some of those techniques later in this chapter.

Exercise: Keeping a Food Diary

Here's a blank food diary for your own use. (A downloadable version of this form, which you can use to keep a food diary over time, is available at http://www.newharbinger .com/31304; see the back of the book for information on how to access it.) Use this form to monitor your daily food and beverage intake for four of the next seven days. It's best to choose three days during the week and one weekend day, as people tend to eat and drink differently on the weekends than during the week.

Food Diary

Breakfast (amount and type of food or drink)	Calories

Lunch (amount and type of food or drink)	Calories

Dinner (amount and type of food or drink)	Calories

Snacks (amount and type of food or drink)	Calories
Total calories for the day	

The Challenges of Keeping a Food Diary

Given that you're reading this book on wellness, you're probably interested in changing your diet—perhaps because you're eating and drinking more often than you'd like to throughout your day. It's also possible that you're eating many meals out, rather than going to the grocery store and cooking your own meals, given that having a mood disorder can make these tasks more challenging (Kilbourne et al. 2007). This will make monitoring your daily food consumption difficult, since you probably won't know how restaurant foods were prepared. You may also notice that when you're depressed or manic, it's also more difficult to take the time to fill out your food diary each day. Many people with bipolar disorder feel this way, so take heart from knowing that you are not alone. Here's an example of someone struggling with this very problem.

> George works in the city, doesn't like to cook, and loves Italian food. So he usually eats lunch, and often dinner, at Italian restaurants near his workplace. Recently, George went to his doctor for his annual checkup and found out he has high cholesterol. His doctor suggested that he monitor his diet carefully to reduce his cholesterol levels, and George left the appointment very motivated to change his diet. It was lunchtime and he was hungry, so he decided to stop at one of his favorite restaurants on his way back to work.
>
> George ordered a typical meal for him: chicken marsala, a side of pasta with red sauce, and a cannoli for dessert. While eating, he pulled out the food diary his doctor had given him and tried to record the components of his meal. He wrote "chicken," but then felt confused because he didn't know what was in the marsala sauce. So he moved on and wrote "pasta," but he wasn't sure how much pasta he was eating. Was it just 1 cup or maybe 2? As for the cannoli, he had no idea what was in it. By the time he finished his meal, George decided that he simply couldn't record everything he ate. As a result, George thought that he was a failure.

Does this story sound familiar? It's understandable that people sometimes become overwhelmed by the task of writing down all of the components of everything they eat and the amount of each, especially when eating out. Keeping an accurate food diary isn't easy. It can take a lot of willpower (not to mention honesty!) to write down each thing you eat, down to every single snack. It can also take a lot of brainpower to remember what you've consumed and how much. If you find that you lack the willpower or desire to keep an accurate food diary, refer back to chapter 1 and revisit how you can get out of the contemplation stage of change and into the preparation and action stage. I'll also review a few other ways to increase your motivation to keep a food diary later in this chapter. Then, in the next chapter, we'll look at how to handle those overly negative thoughts about failing.

If you find that you're having difficulty with the brainpower part of keeping a food diary—remembering what you consume and the serving sizes of everything—try some problem-solving strategies. Here are a few that might be helpful, with some examples based on George's experience to make the suggestions clearer:

- Use the "Visual Guide to Serving Sizes" earlier in this chapter. This could help George estimate how much pasta and chicken he ate.

- Find nutritional information for complicated foods (like sauces) online or with an app. For example, George could search for "nutritional information for marsala sauce." The information he finds might not be exactly the same as for the restaurant's marsala sauce, but it will probably provide a good approximation. Knowing the nutritional content of something like a prepared sauce is the goal, so it isn't necessary to write down each ingredient in these kinds of foods.

- Consider eating out less frequently. Serving sizes of restaurant foods and their calorie content can be difficult to assess, and the food at restaurants may not be very nutritious, given that they typically aim for foods that are tasty, regardless of fat content or empty calories. In George's case, even though he doesn't like to cook, he could look to find ways to make cooking easier such as buying healthy frozen or prepared foods at the store. He could also choose restaurants with healthier food options or only eat half of his meal and bring the rest home.

- Keep older food diaries on hand as a source of information. Once George figures out and records the foods, portion sizes, and calories in this meal, he can just reference that information next time he has any of the components of that meal.

- Start slowly. As you learned in chapter 2, it's important to set realistic goals, including in regard to monitoring your diet, so that you don't feel tempted to quit. If George feels overwhelmed at the thought of keeping a food diary daily, or even four days per week, he could begin by recording his breakfast and lunch four days per week, or he might record everything he consumes for two full days the first week.

- Start keeping a food diary with a friend. George might not have become so overwhelmed if he'd had a friend there to help him, or maybe he would have stuck with it if he'd agreed to share completed food diaries with a friend each week.

- Keep the ultimate goal in mind. George isn't monitoring his diet just for the sake of doing so, or even to lose weight. His ultimate goal is to protect his health by reducing his cholesterol levels. If he reminds himself of this, it might provide motivation to monitor his diet and begin to improve it.

- Identify obstacles and figure out how to overcome them. If George were to write down all of the reasons he has trouble completing his food diaries, he could do some problem solving.

The last strategy in that list—identifying obstacles and figuring out how to overcome them—is extremely helpful. It's also an approach that you can apply to many different areas of life, so it's a skill well worth learning. The next exercise will guide you through how to do this.

Exercise: Overcoming Obstacles to Keeping a Food Diary

The following worksheet covers some of the most common obstacles to keeping a food diary, along with potential solutions. It also includes blank spaces for you to record other obstacles you may face and your ideas about solutions to those problems. If you have trouble identifying your obstacles, you may want to try keeping a food diary for a few days to understand what your obstacles are.

When using the worksheet, check the box to the left of the "Obstacle" column if you think the obstacle listed in that row might be a challenge for you. Then read the possible solutions in the right-hand column.

The solutions listed here are just for your guidance; try to think of things that have worked in the past to help you be successful at completing other challenging tasks. Everyone usually has some unique solutions that work just for them. Be creative! I once had a client tell me that he wore green socks on the days he intended to keep a food diary to remind him to do it. If something works, it's generally a good solution.

Problem-Solving Worksheet for Completing Food Diaries

✔	Obstacle	Possible solutions
☐	Lack of motivation or energy	• Review your rationale for completing a food diary. • Give yourself a reward, such as having a favorite beverage, for completing your food diary. • Ask a friend to keep a food diary too. • Refer back to your behavioral analysis (see chapter 1) to see what you identified as coping skills during that exercise. • Other:
☐	Lack of interest	• Review your rationale for completing a food diary. • Try an experiment: Complete your food diary for two days to see if doing so helps you be more aware of what you're eating and drinking. If so, remind yourself that this is the first step to making changes and becoming more healthy. • Try a different technique. If you started with a written diary, switch to an electronic format, and vice versa. • Complete a thought record (described later in this chapter) to help change your thinking about food diaries. • Other:
☐	Forgetting to do it	• Write down each food and beverage right after you consume it. • Keep your food diary with you. • Set a reminder on your phone or write yourself a note and post it someplace obvious. • Complete your food diary at the same time every day. • Other:

✔	Obstacle	Possible solutions
☐	Not wanting to take the time	• Consider an alternative strategy to a written food diary, such as an online program or phone app. • Keep a log of your most common meals so you have the information for each readily available. • Remind yourself of your rationale for keeping a food diary. • Other:
☐	Feeling guilty about foods or beverages consumed	• Complete a thought record (described later in this chapter) to help change your thinking. • Remind yourself that being aware of what you're eating is the first step in changing your diet. • Remind yourself that most people underestimate how much they're eating, so you are not alone. • Get support from a friend or family member. • Other:
☐	Other:	
☐	Other:	
☐	Other:	

Changing Your Thinking

A common obstacle to making lifestyle changes is having negative automatic thoughts. By *automatic thoughts*, I mean immediate, spontaneous thoughts that come to mind during certain situations. They may be about yourself, the world, other people, or the future. They tend to arise quickly and in rapid succession, without you consciously bringing them to mind, especially during emotionally challenging events.

In regard to food diaries, these might include thoughts such as *Keeping a food diary won't help me, I'll never have the time to keep a food diary, My diet is too unhealthy and it makes me feel awful to see it written down,* or *I've tried to change my diet before and failed; I'll never be able to maintain a healthy lifestyle.* Remember, having bipolar disorder means that you're more likely to have these kinds of negative thoughts. There is good news, though: Thoughts aren't necessarily accurate or correct. They can be wrong, inaccurate, or otherwise distorted.

It's typical that most of a person's thoughts are just assumptions about things. And importantly, when people are upset, stressed, or in a bad mood, including being depressed or manic, their assumptions may be overly negative or less likely to be accurate. Although everyone is prone to making false assumptions (or other thinking errors), people with bipolar disorder tend to have more false assumptions and to be more likely to believe that these assumptions are correct.

There's actually a silver lining to this: It's possible to work on your false assumptions to create more accurate thoughts. And if you have many negative assumptions, when you change them you'll end up with many thoughts that are more positive or accurate. This will go a long way toward increasing your feelings of well-being on a day-to-day basis.

As to how to change your thinking, it's essentially a four-step process:

1. Identify negative automatic thoughts.

2. Distinguish which are false assumptions, rather than facts (something I'll cover at length in chapter 6).

3. Examine the evidence against your false assumptions.

4. Generate new, alternative thoughts.

The following sections will guide you through the process. Then, because this is such a key skill, we'll revisit the topic in chapter 6.

Identifying Automatic Thoughts

Identifying automatic thoughts can be tricky because they're just so…automatic. When they arise, they may just feel "right," making it tempting to assume they're true. However, a set of key questions can help you distinguish which thoughts are automatic. To see how they work, let's consider an example.

Lisa lives with her mother and has difficulty getting along with her. One Saturday, Lisa's mother asked her why she wasn't going out with friends that night. Lisa became very upset because she thought it wasn't any of her mother's business what she did on the weekends. But then Lisa started thinking that she didn't have any friends she could call to go out with, which made her sad. Ultimately, she started thinking about how she seemed to be stuck living with her mom and had no friends, and ended up feeling like she'd never be able to get out of her current situation, which made her angry. Ultimately, Lisa decided to spend that Saturday night alone in her bedroom, watching movies and snacking on junk food.

Now let's take a look at how Lisa might use the key questions below to identify her automatic thoughts. For each question, I've provided potential automatic thoughts; you might have ideas about others.

What went through my mind first? *I have no one to go out with this weekend.*

What do these thoughts mean about me? *I have no friends.*

What do these thoughts mean about me in the big picture (for my life and my future)? *I'm a loser because I live at home with my mother and have no friends.*

What do I fear might happen if these thoughts are true? *I'll always be alone, and I'll keep stuffing my face when I'm lonely, so I'll always be overweight.*

What's the worst thing that could happen if these thoughts are true? *I'll die alone and never be healthy again.*

What do these thoughts suggest in terms of what other people might think or feel about me? *People will think I'm a loser because I'll be overweight and alone.*

What do these thoughts mean about other people in general? *Other people seem to be able to make friends and lose weight. Other people are better than me.*

As you can see, Lisa's brief interaction with her mother triggered a complex set of thoughts about being alone on a Saturday night. Imagine if you had these thoughts; you might also feel bad about yourself and choose to isolate yourself and overeat. However, do you think all of Lisa's thoughts are true or 100 percent accurate? Chances are, Lisa actually has at least a few friends or knows people who could become friends. So will she really *never* have any friends or *always* be alone on Saturday nights? Likewise, is it true that she'll *never* be able to lose weight? I hope you're seeing that some of Lisa's thoughts are false assumptions. And as you can see, these kinds of thoughts can be overly negative. Worse, they can lead to unhealthy behaviors, despite being false. So everybody needs to work on changing these kinds of thoughts.

Using Evidence to Challenge Assumptions

Once you've identified automatic negative thoughts, you need to consider whether they're factual. In many cases, they aren't, such as in Lisa's example. So look for evidence that contradicts these thoughts. If you find it, you'll know you're dealing with false assumptions. For instance, if you think you don't have time to keep a food diary, you could come up with examples of other situations where you made time for something important to you, or you could review your daily schedule to identify moments of spare time or activities that are less meaningful to you than keeping a food diary.

Finding evidence against your false assumptions can be challenging if you strongly believe these thoughts to be true. If you have difficulty with this, consider seeking support from a trusted friend, family member, or therapist. Once you've identified overly negative thoughts and gathered evidence against them, the next step is to replace them with new, more positive thoughts—a skill known as *cognitive restructuring*. The next exercise will help you begin to develop this skill.

Exercise: Using Evidence to Generate Alternative Thoughts

This exercise will help you weigh the evidence against some common negative thoughts about healthy eating—all of which are false assumptions. After considering the evidence against each thought, you'll practice generating new, alternative thoughts. The negative thoughts I've provided here are things I've heard from clients with bipolar disorder over the years. Some of them may seem familiar to you, and when you read them, you may find yourself thinking, *But healthy foods are expensive!* While there may be some truth in this, are *all* healthy foods expensive? And do you perhaps find it easier to spend money on expensive but *un*healthy foods that you really like?

All of the thoughts below tend to interfere with people's ability to choose healthy foods. So to the extent that you have any of these thoughts, this exercise will help you overcome obstacles to choosing healthier alternatives, in addition to giving you practice in generating alternative thoughts.

Take some time to read through the following thoughts. For each, come up with some evidence to challenge the thought. Then come up with an alternative thought that supports making changes to eat more healthfully. I've filled out the first one to help you see how it works. I've also provided a couple of blanks so you can work on any other unhelpful thoughts you may have about eating well.

Assumption 1: Healthy foods are expensive.

Evidence against this thought: *I know that there are some common fruits and vegetables that aren't that pricey. I can also buy leaner meat, which is more expensive, in bulk and freeze what I won't use right away for later. That would save money. Plus, I seem to find the money to buy expensive, unhealthy foods, so I know I can afford to buy some foods that are healthier.*

Alternative thought 1: *Some healthy foods can be expensive, but there are many choices that are cheap and still healthy.*

Assumption 2: I can no longer eat my favorite foods if I diet.

Evidence against this thought: _____

_____

_____

Alternative thought 2: _____

_____

Assumption 3: I deserve to treat myself with unhealthy foods.

Evidence against this thought: _____

_____

_____

Alternative thought 3: _____

_____

Assumption 4: My medications cause weight gain.

Evidence against this thought: _____

_____

_____

Alternative thought 4: _____

_____

Assumption 5: Eating healthy takes too much effort.

Evidence against this thought: _____

_____

_____

Alternative thought 5: _____

_____

Assumption 6: _____

Evidence against this thought: _____

_____

_____

Alternative thought 6: _____

_____

Assumption 7: _____

Evidence against this thought: _____

_____

_____

Alternative thought 7: _____

_____

How did that go? Could you readily come up with evidence against these assumptions? How difficult was it to come up with new, alternative thoughts? Some people have a little more trouble with the fourth assumption: *My medications cause weight gain*. If that was the case for you, here's some evidence against it: Medications can increase your cravings for certain foods, but they don't make you gain weight. Weight gain happens when people eat too much or don't exercise enough, and those are both things a person can control. Based on that evidence, you might consider having another go at coming up with an alternative to the fourth assumption.

Exercise: Keeping a Thought Record

A thought record is a very useful tool for changing your thinking. In brief, this process involves describing the situation—the facts about the event—then recording your thoughts or perceptions about the event. Next, you identify the emotions those thoughts and perceptions trigger and rate their intensity. Then you come up with an alternative thought—one that's supported by evidence—and assess how the intensity of each emotion changes.

In this chapter, I'll provide detailed instructions for completing a thought record, followed by a blank worksheet for your use. But first, here's a sample worksheet to help you see how it works.

Sample Thought Record Worksheet

Situation	Who	Me
	What	Feeling bad about eating a lot of junk food today
	Where	At home
	When	Monday, 9 p.m.

Automatic thoughts	Emotions (0–10)	Alternative thoughts	Emotions (0–10)
I didn't eat well today.	Guilt (8)	It's important to eat well, but it won't help me to get mad at myself for not eating well today.	Guilt (4)
I'll never be able to eat well or change my diet.	Fear (9)	I know that I can change my diet because I've made other changes, such as making a new friend despite being very anxious in social situations.	Fear (6)
I'll gain weight and continue to have high cholesterol.	Fear (7)	I need to make changes to my diet, and I can learn from why I didn't eat well today so that I can eat better tomorrow.	Fear (3)
People will think that I'm lazy for not taking better care of my health.	Fear (9)	I'm not a lazy person. I do many other things, such as work hard at my job and pay my bills.	Fear (1)
I'll never find a partner.	Sadness (10)	A good partner will love me regardless of my weight. I also know that overweight people find partners.	Sadness (2)
I'll be alone.	Sadness (10) Fear (10)	I'm not alone; I have friends and family.	Sadness (3) Fear (2)

> **Questions to help identify automatic thoughts:**
>
> What went through my mind just as I thought about the situation?
>
> What do these thoughts mean about me?
>
> What do these thoughts mean about me in the big picture (for my life and my future)?
>
> What do I fear might happen if these thoughts are true?
>
> What's the worst thing that could happen if these thoughts are true?
>
> What do these thoughts suggest in terms of what other people might think or feel about me?
>
> What do these thoughts mean about other people in general?

Situation

Now that you have the example to refer to, let's go through the worksheet section by section. The rows at the top are for describing the situation ("Who," "What," "Where," and "When"). In this section, it's very important to focus only on the facts. It can be all too easy to interpret the event, applying automatic thoughts to it even when just describing it. To stay focused on an objective description of the event, ask yourself the four Ws:

Who was involved in the situation?

What happened during the situation?

Where did the situation occur?

When did it happen?

These questions can usually be answered with just a few words, as you can see in the sample worksheet.

Automatic Thoughts

Then, in the left-hand column under "Automatic thoughts," write down all of the automatic thoughts that came up in the situation. Your thoughts may also wander to other situations, especially if you're currently hypomanic or manic and experiencing racing thoughts. Try to stay focused only on the situation you're looking at in the thought record.

Emotions Triggered by Automatic Thoughts

In the next column ("Emotions"), record the emotions triggered by each automatic thought. Try to stick with basic emotions in this column, such as "sadness," "loneliness," "fear," "guilt," "jealousy," "anger," "frustration," or "shame." As you may notice, the emotions listed are all on the unpleasant side; that's because this exercise is for analyzing thoughts that are difficult or troublesome.

Also, be aware that people often say things like "I feel stupid" or "I feel disrespected," but these statements are actually thoughts that you're having, not feelings or emotions. You may *think* that you're stupid or disrespected, but this may not be true, so it can't be a feeling or emotion. Feelings and emotions are *always* true or correct because they reflect your mood, which is just the way you feel at any given time. Thoughts, on the other hand, are judgments or interpretations of your environment. So be sure to distinguish between feelings and thoughts. You may well be able to change your thoughts. In fact, that's exactly the goal here—to work on changing negative thoughts while accepting your feelings without judgment. To be clear, by "accepting," I don't mean you have to like or embrace your emotions; you simply need to be aware of them and allow them to arise and then recede, as they eventually will.

After identifying the emotions a thought brings up, rate the intensity of that emotion on a scale of 0 to 10, with 10 being the most strongly you've ever felt that emotion and 0 being a total absence of that emotion.

Alternative Thoughts

In the third column ("Alternative thoughts"), you'll write new thoughts based on evidence that contradicts the automatic thought. For example, in the sample worksheet you can see that this person thinks eating junk food will make her gain weight. There may be some truth to this thought; eating junk food on a regular basis can lead to weight gain for many people. But will just one day of bingeing on junk food make a person fat? No. This is the key: you need to focus on each situation individually. You may have a day when you don't eat well, but this doesn't mean you're incapable of changing your diet. That is just another overly negative thought.

Instead, look for alternative thoughts that support the healthy lifestyle changes you'd like to make, such as *I know I can change my diet because I've done it before* or *I know I can change my diet because I've been successful at making other changes in my life*. Other possible alternative thoughts might be *I can learn from why it was difficult for me to eat well today and use what I learn to make better decisions tomorrow*.

A key point about alternative thoughts is that they usually aren't either overly positive (*Not eating well is fine; it won't make me gain weight*) or overly negative (*I'm an awful person if I don't eat well all the time*). So try to come up with alternative thoughts that are balanced or realistic. This may be challenging to do on your own, especially if you really believe your automatic thoughts. Consider having someone help you brainstorm alternative thoughts. Another helpful strategy is to pretend that your automatic thoughts are someone else's. What would you tell a friend about eating too much junk food one day? This approach will help you distance yourself emotionally from your automatic thoughts so you can look at them more objectively.

Emotions Triggered by Alternative Thoughts

Finally, in the right-hand column, for each alternative thought write the same emotions as in the second column (for your automatic thought), then rate the intensity of each emotion after considering the alternative thought. If you've come up with effective alternative thoughts, you should notice that your ratings are lower. If the intensity of your emotions has stayed the same or increased, your alternative thoughts aren't effectively challenging your automatic thoughts. You need to go back and generate new alternative thoughts.

Now that you understand how to complete a thought record, here's a blank worksheet for your use. (For a downloadable version of this worksheet, which you can use to work with other difficult situations, visit http://www.newharbinger.com/31304. See the back of the book for instructions on how to access the worksheet.)

Start simple, with automatic thoughts that are less emotionally intense. You might choose a situation such as being stuck in traffic, being frustrated about the weather, or having to watch TV commercials. You have thoughts in every situation, so start with simple situations. That will help you get the hang of this process before you apply it to intense thoughts, perhaps about your weight, health, or difficulty exercising.

Thought Record Worksheet

Situation		
	Who	
	What	
	Where	
	When	

Automatic thoughts	Emotions (0–10)	Alternative thoughts	Emotions (0–10)

Questions to help identify automatic thoughts:
What went through my mind just as I thought about the situation?
What do these thoughts mean about me?
What do these thoughts mean about me in the big picture (for my life and my future)?
What do I fear might happen if these thoughts are true?
What's the worst thing that could happen if these thoughts are true?
What do these thoughts suggest in terms of what other people might think or feel about me?
What do these thoughts mean about other people in general?

I recommend completing a thought record several times each week to help you practice changing your thinking. As you get more experience with cognitive restructuring, start choosing situations in which you did something that was contrary to the goals you identified in chapter 2. For example, perhaps you planned to increase your activity level on a certain day by going for a walk, but you ended up watching TV instead. To get started, ask yourself the questions that can help identify automatic thoughts, which appear at the end of the worksheet. Focus on the specific time when you decided not to go for the walk and stay inside instead. What went through your mind at that time?

The Brain Is Always Thinking

I find that a common stumbling block in completing thought records is that people have difficulty identifying automatic thoughts. They often say they don't have any thoughts when engaging in problem behaviors, like overeating, not exercising, or other activities that promote an unhealthy lifestyle. But is it really possible to have no thoughts in any situation? No, it isn't, even in the most cut-and-dried situation. For example, if you're walking across the street and see a car coming, you may run out of the way. It might seem that you're just reacting without thinking, but you must have had the thought that a car was coming in order to pick up your pace in crossing the street. In short, to act we must think.

We always have thoughts, whether while eating "mindlessly," watching TV, or "doing nothing." These thoughts may be as simple as *This tastes good*, *That's funny*, or *I don't have anything to do right now*. The fact is, if you believe you aren't having any thoughts in a given situation, you're actually just having trouble identifying thoughts, because we *always* have thoughts. I recommend that you practice observing your automatic thoughts in situations where you're more aware of your thoughts. Later, this will help you identify your automatic thoughts at times when it might initially seem as though you don't have any thoughts.

Practice, Practice, Practice

Changing our thinking is a very powerful tool. Researchers have found that this can actually change how the brain functions (for example, Goldapple et al. 2004). This is particularly important for people with bipolar disorder, a disease in which brain cells aren't functioning properly. However, cognitive restructuring is only effective when you actually *practice* using the alternative thoughts you generate, so take some time to read through your new, alternative thoughts and actively think about them every day. Here's a way of looking at it that may help you see how this can help.

Imagine that your overly negative thoughts, which tend to pop up quickly and frequently, are like water flowing downstream in a river. The more negative thoughts you have, the more water you have, and the faster and harder the river flows… Now imagine that your alternative, more objective and positive thoughts are branches you place in the river. For every alternative thought you have, you place another branch in the river. If you identify a lot of these alternative, positive thoughts and think of them often, you'll have a lot of branches in the river. This will slow the speed of the current (your negative thoughts). If you add enough branches, you may even be able to stop the flow.

However, if you don't actively think of these alternative thoughts *every day*, the branches are likely to wash away. The river of your negative thoughts will pick up speed again, making it harder to put those branches back and stop the flow. In short, thinking positive alternative thoughts is an active process. You have to work at putting those branches in the river. So in the end, changing your thinking requires not only that you identify new thoughts, but also that you then make sure you think them frequently—at least as often as you think the negative thoughts. Initially, it may feel odd to intentionally repeat new, positive thoughts over and over again in your head, especially if you're having trouble believing these new thoughts. Stick with it! Eventually, you'll see a change in your thinking.

That said, if you have difficulty practicing your new thoughts, the problem may simply be that you haven't identified the right alternative thoughts for you. Alternative thoughts are often called *coping thoughts* because they should help you cope with difficult situations. If, after practicing your new thoughts repeatedly for a few weeks, they still don't help you cope, you probably need to generate some new alternatives. Again, this is particularly important for you; because you have bipolar disorder, your river of negative thoughts probably flows very fast quite often, so you need to have strong branches—effective alternative thoughts—to slow this stream of negative thinking.

Exercise: Using Coping Cards

An obstacle to practicing your new, alternative thoughts—or to using them in difficult situations—can be simply not remembering to do so. If that's the case for you, coping cards can be helpful. The name "coping cards" came about because originally index cards were used to record coping thoughts. There are various ways to make coping cards (outlined briefly in the pages that follow), but the key is to record ways to cope with challenges to making healthy lifestyle choices—including remembering your alternative thoughts. Whatever form they take, keep your coping cards with you at all times. To help you remember the rationale for your new coping thoughts, I recommend that you write a coping thought on one side of a card, if you're using one, and record your strategies for helping you act on your new thought on the other side. Here are some examples:

Front of card	Back of card
Some foods can taste good and still be healthy.	• Choices that are tasty *and* healthy include grapes, low-fat yogurt, popcorn, ice pops, fish, chicken, low-fat meat, Cheerios, and whole grain English muffins. • There are many healthy foods that I still need to try, such as hummus. • I can remind myself that even though unhealthy foods sometimes taste better, I usually don't feel well after I eat them.
I can make changes to my diet to eat healthier, low-calorie foods.	• I can snack on popcorn or baked chips instead of fried potato chips. • I can remind myself that I feel better after eating healthier foods. • I can motivate myself with small rewards, like watching a funny clip on YouTube, when I make healthy food choices. • Eating meals with a healthy friend can help me learn to eat better.
I can eat more fruits and vegetables.	• I like many fruits and vegetables, such as cherries, pineapple, bananas, green beans, and carrots. • I can have a salad with fruit for one meal, and it could include two servings each of fruits and vegetables. • I can buy frozen fruits and vegetables, which are cheaper and keep longer.

If you have a smartphone, it may be easier to record your new thoughts, along with strategies for acting on them or evidence supporting them, in a notes app on your phone. Alternatively, you could set up reminders with your coping thoughts so that they pop up on your phone regularly—every day, or even every hour of every day. This is especially important for people who have bipolar disorder, since bipolar disorder can make it more difficult to remember things. The point is, if you enjoy technology, use it to help you practice your new thoughts and act on them. But if you prefer written reminders, that's fine too. Index cards remain a great choice because they're small and convenient—which is important, because you want your new, alternative thoughts, the evidence for them, and strategies for acting on them to be close at hand and easily accessible.

Summary

- Monitoring your food and beverage consumption is important for eating healthier and losing weight.

- There can be many obstacles to tracking your daily diet. Identifying them is the first step in figuring out how to overcome them.

- One major obstacle is having overly negative thoughts or false assumptions about keeping a food diary or about your diet.

- A thought record can help you change negative thoughts and come up with new, alternative thoughts.

- Coping cards are useful for remembering and practicing your alternative thoughts and starting to act on them.

Chapter 5

Understanding the
Power of Activity

In chapters 3 and 4, we looked at the role of dietary choices in creating a healthy lifestyle. Your wellness depends on good nutrition, eating a balanced diet, and eating an appropriate amount of food—all crucial aspects of a healthy lifestyle. But exercise is equally important for your mental and physical health. So, in this chapter and the next, we'll examine physical activity and how it can not only benefit your physical health, but also ease your symptoms of bipolar disorder.

Why Exercise for Bipolar Disorder?

You may remember from chapter 1 that people with bipolar disorder are more likely than other people to have risk factors for cardiovascular disease, such as being overweight, having high blood pressure, or having high cholesterol levels (Soreca, Frank, and Kupfer 2009). This can be discouraging, especially when added to the challenges you face in managing your bipolar symptoms, such as sad mood, fatigue, difficulty concentrating, or irritability. Yet there's also some good news. There is a non-medication-based treatment that can help reduce your risk of both cardiovascular disease *and* your bipolar symptoms. This treatment is exercise.

You probably aren't shocked to hear that exercising can help you lose weight and keep weight off, and also lower your cholesterol and blood pressure levels, but did you know that exercise can also help with depression? As mentioned in chapter 1, one study of people with unipolar depression found that exercising three days per week, for forty-five minutes each time, over a four-month period was as effective in improving depressive symptoms as sertraline, an antidepressant medication (Blumenthal et al. 1999; Babyak et al. 2000). Another study, this one conducted with people who had bipolar disorder, found that those who walked just eight times, for thirty minutes each time, had a more positive outlook on life and that stress tended to bother them less than usual (Edenfield 2008).

Scientists are beginning to understand the mechanisms in the body that allow exercise to improve the symptoms of depression. This is very exciting because it further confirms that exercise is a powerful intervention for depression. For example, recent data indicates that exercise spurs the growth of new brain cells, a process called *neurogenesis* (Duman 2005; Ernst et al. 2006). Neurogenesis is important because it improves the brain's ability to adapt to things, which helps with stress management. It also benefits other brain functions, such as learning and memory, including consolidation and storage of memories (Lu 2003; Binder and Scharfman 2004).

Exercise and Mania

The potential benefits of exercise for the elevated mood states in bipolar disorder—hypomania and mania—aren't as clear. Although some people with bipolar disorder believe that exercise helps regulate mood swings in general or has a calming effect, it may be a double-edged sword, sometimes having harmful effects on the symptoms of bipolar disorder (Wright et al. 2012). For example, my colleagues and I recently found that exercise is associated with more manic symptoms; however, it's unclear whether exercise is causing mania or people who are manic are just exercising more (Sylvia, Friedman, et al. 2013). For now, it's probably best to assume that people may have an individualized response to exercise when they're in a hypomanic or manic state. For some people it may help, and for others it may not. It's important to pay attention to your own experience and be cautious about starting an exercise program when you're manic or hypomanic, or if you believe that you may become manic or hypomanic soon. In these situations, it may be advisable to talk with your doctor before making major changes in your activity level.

Why Everyone Should Exercise

Of course, exercise has numerous benefits for everyone, not just people with bipolar disorder. And because the goal of this workbook is to help you improve your overall wellness, all of these benefits are important for you. You may be well acquainted with how exercise can improve your health. Still, this information can be very motivating, so let's take a quick look at some of the most important ways in which exercise benefits both physical and mental health.

Sleep. Studies have shown that exercise can improve the quality and duration of sleep and the ease of falling asleep. This may occur because exercise reduces stress, warms the body, and relaxes the muscles (Yang et al. 2012). Sleep is particularly important for people with bipolar disorder, given that not sleeping well has been shown to worsen bipolar symptoms (Ng et al. 2014). For this reason, almost anything that promotes sleep, including exercise, has been considered a treatment strategy for bipolar disorder (Ravindran and da Silva 2013).

Anxiety. Brisk walking or running often improves anxiety symptoms, particularly among people with anxiety disorders (Wegner et al. 2014). This has a bearing on bipolar disorder because many people with bipolar disorder also have an anxiety disorder. So if you have bipolar disorder and experience anxiety, exercise could be very helpful. One reason is that exercise reduces anxiety sensitivity, or the likelihood that you'll perceive things as being anxiety provoking. Exercise also causes physiological changes that can reduce your anxiety, such as boosting the production of hormones and neurotransmitters (brain chemicals) that help balance your mood.

Smoking. Exercise is also associated with reduced cravings to smoke cigarettes and may ease nicotine withdrawal symptoms (Fong et al. 2014). I mention smoking in particular because some studies have shown that nearly half the people with bipolar disorder smoke regularly (Heffner et al. 2013). So you are not alone if you struggle with these cravings. If you do smoke, consider exercising as a way to help you quit. As an added bonus, exercise can also make it easier to decrease use of other substances, such as alcohol (Zschucke, Heinz, and Ströhle 2012).

Memory. Both aerobic exercise and strength training have been associated with cognitive benefits (Weinberg et al. 2014). As mentioned previously, people with bipolar disorder are likely to have more difficulty remembering things; this is simply one of the characteristics of the illness (Buoli et al. 2014). Imagine how great it would be to have an inexpensive treatment that could help you think and focus better. Exercise is that treatment!

Physical health improvements. Last but certainly not least, exercise can improve physical health in so many ways, helping prevent many serious medical conditions, including heart disease. Exercise increases the supply of oxygen to the heart muscle by expanding existing blood vessels and creating tiny new blood vessels. It may also prevent blood clots or promote their breakdown (Stoner et al. 2012). This also reduces blood pressure if it's high or helps maintain a healthy blood pressure level (Arroll and Beaglehole 1992). Exercise also helps to reduce the risk of developing diabetes, especially among those who are already at risk because of obesity, high blood pressure, or a family history of diabetes (Hu et al. 1999). Finally, regular moderate exercise (either aerobic or strength training) can reduce joint swelling and pain in people with arthritis (Ettinger et al. 1997).

Let's Rename Exercise!

Given all of those benefits, it seems exercising regularly would be a no-brainer—something everyone would want to do. Yet clearly this isn't the case, especially among people with bipolar disorder, perhaps due to the fatigue and lack of interest and motivation, which are common symptoms of depression. Many of my clients claim that they just can't exercise. Here's a fairly typical example.

> Bob used to exercise a lot when he was younger. He was on his high school track-and-field team and says he used to love to run. In college he kept running on his own for a few years because he enjoyed it and wanted to stay in shape, but in his senior year he started experiencing symptoms of depression. He felt tired all the time, had a sad mood, and started having trouble sleeping, which often left him irritable and angry. Before the year was over, he stopped running. Several years later, when he came to me for therapy, he reported that he had several periodic episodes of depression every year and a hypomanic or manic episode about once a year. He'd gained weight since college and wasn't happy about it, but he said he felt that exercise was too much for him now. I asked him to define exercise, and he said "running three or four times a week."

That seems like a lot of exercise, especially for someone who's been mostly inactive for a few years. Do you think it might be hard to go from not exercising at all to doing a high-intensity form of exercise, such as running, every other day? I certainly do.

As a result of so many similar conversations with clients, I now advocate renaming "exercise" as "lifestyle activity." My definition of *lifestyle activity* includes exercise of any intensity, whether low or high. After all, any form of exercise or movement can have positive benefits for your mind and body. The term "lifestyle activity" also serves as a reminder that any type of activity, whether an organized sport, such as basketball or track and field, or daily activities, like housecleaning or walking up stairs, counts toward a healthy lifestyle.

I think switching to the term "lifestyle activity" is particularly important for people with bipolar disorder, given the likelihood of having more frequent and intense negative thoughts about exercising. So let's start thinking about exercise differently. Give yourself credit for any activity that gets your body in motion and burns more calories. In the end, it's making an important contribution to improving your mental and physical health.

If you have any doubts about that, take a look at the following table, which outlines the number of calories burned by doing various activities for ten minutes. As you can see, an activity like getting dressed can burn practically as many calories as mild exercise, such as walking at 2 miles per hour, and many chores, such as making beds or weeding, burn more calories than slow walking. And you may be surprised to see that walking up stairs actually burns more calories than running at 7 miles per hour.

Calories Burned in 10 Minutes of Activity

Activity		Body weight		
		125 lbs	175 lbs	250 lbs
Personal necessities	Sleeping	10	14	20
	Sitting	10	14	18
	Dressing or washing	26	37	53
	Standing	12	16	24

Activity		Body weight		
		125 lbs	175 lbs	250 lbs
Locomotion	Walking downstairs	56	78	111
	Walking upstairs	146	202	288
	Walking at 2 mph	29	40	58
	Walking at 4 mph	52	72	102
	Running at 5.5 mph	90	125	178
	Running at 7 mph	118	164	232
	Cycling at 5.5 mph	42	58	83
	Cycling at 13 mph	89	124	178
Housework	Making beds	32	46	65
	Washing floors	38	53	75
	Washing windows	35	48	69
	Dusting	22	31	44
	Preparing a meal	32	46	65
	Shoveling snow	65	89	130
	Light gardening	30	42	59
	Weeding garden	49	68	98
	Mowing grass	34	47	67
Sedentary work	Typing on computer	19	27	39
	Light office work	25	34	50
	Standing, light activity	20	28	40
Light work	Assembly line	20	28	40
	Auto repair	35	48	69
	Carpentry	32	44	64
	Bricklaying	28	40	57
	Farming chores	32	44	64
	House painting	29	40	58

Heavy work	Pick and shovel work	56	78	110
	Chopping wood	60	84	121
	Dragging logs	158	220	315
Recreation	Badminton	43	65	94
	Baseball	39	54	78
	Basketball	58	82	117
	Bowling (nonstop)	56	78	111
	Canoeing (4 mph)	90	128	182
	Dancing (moderate)	35	48	69
	Dancing (vigorous)	48	66	94
	Football	69	96	137
	Golfing	33	48	68
	Horseback riding	56	78	112
	Ping-pong	32	45	64
	Racquetball	75	104	144
	Skiing (alpine)	80	112	160
	Skiing (cross country)	98	138	194
	Skiing (water)	60	88	130
	Squash	75	104	144
	Swimming (backstroke)	32	45	64
	Swimming (crawl)	40	56	80
	Tennis	56	80	115
	Volleyball	43	65	94

From Kelly D. Brownell, *The LEARN Program for Weight Management 2000* (Euless, TX: American Health Publishing Company, 2000). Copyright © 2000 Kelly Brownell, PhD. All rights reserved. Used here with permission; other use may be prohibited by law.

Types of Activity

For optimum wellness, you need to engage in several different types of activity: aerobic activites, strength training, and stretching.

Aerobic activities (also known as cardiovascular exercise) utilize large muscle groups and increase the amount of oxygen the body uses. As such, they increase the capacity of the circulatory and respiratory systems to supply oxygen to skeletal muscles, improving cardiovascular fitness. They are typically longer-duration activities. Examples include brisk walking, running, dancing, and cycling.

Strength training (also known as resistance training) is any activity that uses weights or resistance to build muscle mass and strength. It also enhances bone health, among other benefits. It often involves intense, shorter-duration movements. Weight lifting and exercise with resistance bands are obvious examples, but yoga, Pilates, and isometric exercises also fit into this category.

Stretching (also known as flexibility training) is just what you'd imagine: any movements that lengthen muscles. More technically speaking, it's any activity in which specific muscles, muscle groups, or tendons are deliberately flexed or stretched to improve the elasticity and achieve comfortable muscle tone. Stretching has many benefits. In addition to improving flexibility, it increases muscle control and range of motion and improves joint health. Stretching is particularly important as you increase your activity level because it can reduce the likelihood of muscle cramps and decrease risk of injury. Because people have a tendency to skip stretching, I'll provide instructions for a few simple stretches later in the chapter.

How Much Activity?

In 2011, the American College of Sports Medicine published recommendations about the ideal duration, intensity, and frequency of exercise for the average person (Garber et al. 2011). These guidelines recommend 150 minutes of moderate-intensity aerobic exercise per week. This exercise can be 30 to 60 minutes several times per week, or you could do multiple shorter sessions, such as 10 minutes at a time. Either approach is acceptable, as long as you accumulate the recommended 150 minutes of activity weekly.

Regarding strength training, the American College of Sports Medicine suggests that adults do strength-training forms of exercise two to three days per week, and that people start with very light resistance if they haven't done this type of activity before or in a long time.

The American College of Sports Medicine also suggests stretching at least two days per week and holding each stretch for ten to thirty seconds at the point of tightness or slight discomfort. Repeat each stretch two to four times so that you spend at least a minute on each muscle that you're stretching. Stretching is most effective when muscles are warm, so try to do some light aerobic activity or take a warm bath or shower to warm your muscles before stretching.

Here are two other important tips from the American College of Sports Medicine to keep in mind (Garber et al. 2011):

- Increase your exercise duration, frequency, and intensity gradually. This will help reduce your risk of injury and also help you stick to your new activity plan.

- People who are unable to meet the recommendations will still benefit from incorporating more activity into their daily routines.

I suggest speaking with your doctor before beginning to increase your activity level. Your doctor can offer personalized advice on how much activity and which types of activities may work best for you. Your doctor may also provide support and encouragement.

What Is Moderate-Intensity Activity?

The intensity of an aerobic activity is determined by how much energy you burn when doing that activity. It can be measured in units known as *metabolic equivalents* (METs), which are based on your metabolic rate—the rate at which you burn food energy, or calories. The MET of doing any given activity is the ratio of your metabolic rate when doing that activity compared to your metabolic rate when you're at rest. Thus, 1 MET is defined as the energy cost of sitting quietly. For most people, that's equivalent to consumption of about 1 calorie per kilogram of body weight per hour. For a 150-pound person, that would be about 70 calories per hour.

Moderate-intensity exercise is considered to be activity that burns three to six times more calories than when a person is resting, or 3 to 6 METs. These types of activities tend to require a moderate amount of effort and noticeably accelerate your heart rate. Vigorous-intensity exercise is activity that burns more than six times the amount of calories burned at rest, or more than 6 METs. Vigorous activities require a large amount of effort and usually cause rapid breathing and a substantial increase in heart rate.

While it is possible to estimate METs for any given activity, bear in mind that the actual METs for any activity depend on the person and the intensity of effort. Given that caveat, here are some examples of moderate- and vigorous-intensity activities:

Moderate Intensity

- Brisk walking

- Dancing

- Gardening

- Housework

- Playing games and sports with children

- General building tasks, like roofing or painting

- Carrying or moving moderate loads (under forty-five pounds)

Vigorous Intensity

- Running

- Walking briskly uphill

- Fast cycling

- Fast swimming

- Competitive sports, such as football, soccer, or basketball

- Heavy shoveling or digging

- Carrying or moving heavy loads (over forty-five pounds)

How to Get Started

As discussed in chapter 2, when setting goals it's important to choose goals you have a good chance of achieving. You can see the importance of this in Bob's story, earlier in the chapter. Although he hadn't been exercising for several years, as a former track-and-field runner he set the bar too high when he started thinking about increasing his activity level. Rather than choosing small, progressive goals, he set a goal of running three or four times per week. Of course, this didn't work out well for him. Dispirited, he brought it up in our next session:

Bob: I feel like a loser. I totally failed to meet my goal for physical activity.

Dr. Sylvia: Why do you think it's been difficult for you to run three or four times per week?

Bob: It just seems like too much—too overwhelming. I don't think I could run a mile right now.

Dr. Sylvia: Given that we know any type of activity could help you create a healthier life, how else could you increase your level of lifestyle activity?

Bob: Well, I really enjoy walking my dog, Max. So maybe I could do more of that.

Dr. Sylvia: Okay, this sounds like a good idea. How often and how far are you walking Max now? What would you like to set as your new goals in walking Max?

Bob: I walk him every morning, but I usually just get out to the end of my driveway, which is maybe 50 yards long. So maybe a new goal would be to walk him every morning but also at night. I could also try to walk him farther, maybe one mile each time.

Dr. Sylvia: Although I appreciate your enthusiasm to make changes, with these goals you'd be walking about ten times farther than you currently are each day. Does this seem realistic for you to achieve this week?

Bob: I should be able to walk this much, though. After all, I used to be a track-and-field runner! But I do think it would be hard for me to walk so far right away. Maybe I could continue to walk Max every morning but go beyond my driveway to my friend Matt's house, up the street. Maybe I could try walking to Matt's house a few evenings a week too. Or I could walk all the way to my friend Cindy's, at the end of the block.

Dr. Sylvia: It sounds as though you assume you should be able to do everything you did before becoming sick with bipolar disorder. You may be able to, but I wonder if these thoughts of *I should be able to do things* are helpful to you. We can discuss this more later, but for now, your current plan seems much more doable. Maybe you could also talk to Matt about joining you on these walks when you feel ready to go beyond his house.

Based on these and other conversations, Bob and I came up with the following plan to increase his lifestyle activity. Notice how the plan builds upon what Bob is already doing as part of his weekly routine and uses activities that he already enjoys doing, such as walking his dog and going to Matt's house. The first row, the starting point for his plan, outlines Bob's *baseline* activity level: what he's currently doing. Then, each week Bob gradually adds a bit more activity by increasing the number of times he's active, the distance, or the intensity.

Bob's Goal-Setting Worksheet for Getting More Active

Timeline	Plan	Amount of activity
Baseline	*Walk Max to the end of the driveway every morning.*	*7 times/week, 100 yards* *Walk 0.4 miles/week*
Week 1	*Walk Max to Matt's house every morning and two evenings.*	*9 times/week, 200 yards* *Walk 1 mile/week*
Week 2	*Walk Max to Cindy's house every morning and five evenings.*	*12 times/week, 300 yards* *Walk 2 miles/week*
Week 3	*Walk Max to the end of the road two mornings and to Cindy's house the other five mornings and every evening.*	*2 times/week, 0.5 mile* *12 times/week, 300 yards* *Walk 3 miles/week*
Week 4	*Walk Max to the end of the road four mornings and to Cindy's house the other three mornings and every evening.*	*4 times/week, 0.5 mile* *10 times/week, 300 yards* *Walk 3.7 miles/week*
Week 5	*Walk Max to the end of the road every morning and to Cindy's house every evening.*	*7 times/week, 0.5 mile* *7 times/week, 300 yards* *Walk 4.7 miles/week*
Week 6	*Walk Max to the end of the road every morning and two evenings, and to Cindy's house the other five evenings.*	*9 times/week, 0.5 mile* *5 times/week, 300 yards* *Walk 5.4 miles/week*
Week 7	*Walk Max to the end of the road every morning. Jog to Cindy's house two evenings and walk to Cindy's the other five evenings.*	*Walk 4.4 miles/week* *Jog 0.3 mile/week*
Week 8	*Walk Max to the end of the road every morning. Jog to Cindy's house four evenings and walk to Cindy's the other three evenings.*	*Walk 4 miles/week* *Jog 0.7 mile/week*

The preceding dialogue with Bob shows how eager he is to get started on increasing his activity level. Like most people, he wants to get healthier right away. You may feel the same way and aspire to make major changes quickly. Bob also believed he could successfully make big changes because he was very physically active in the past. This is a common trap for people with bipolar disorder: assuming they can do the same things they could do prior to developing the disorder. Bob can certainly get back to running regularly, but it will probably be a bit harder for him to do now because he's experiencing depression.

Keep this in mind as you begin to increase your activity level. You need to be particularly thoughtful about the goals you set. If your goals are too big and therefore difficult to achieve, you may have a hard time building momentum in making changes to your lifestyle. The good news is that once you get started, you're likely to find it easier to keep going, as you begin to experience the many benefits of increasing your activity level.

Exercise: Setting Goals for Increasing Your Activity Level

Now it's time for you to set some goals of your own for increasing your activity level. Bob's example provides great guidance on taking a gradual approach. You might also want to review the tips on goal setting in chapter 2 to make sure you choose goals that are specific and realistic. As far as activities are concerned, that's entirely up to you. At first, you may want to try a variety of activities so you can figure out which ones you enjoy most and which are most suitable or effective for you. The best activity program is one you'll actually stick with, so try to make it fun for yourself.

I've provided a blank eight-week goal-setting worksheet for your use, but you can alter it to use any time frame that works for you. For example, maybe you'd like to plan each day, in which case your plan would extend for just a week or two. Because you'll probably want to continue setting new goals in the months or weeks to come, a downloadable version of this worksheet is available at http://www.newharbinger.com/31304. The downloadable materials also include a one-week, day-by-day worksheet you can use if you prefer to plan your lifestyle activities on a daily basis. See the back of the book for instructions on how to access these downloadable worksheets.

Just to be clear, you don't need to "exercise" every day. In fact, when you're first starting to increase your activity level, it may be best to take every other day off or even just try to increase your activity level one day per week. Giving yourself breaks can be especially important when you're starting out; you don't want to increase your activity level too much too quickly, as this could lead to physical injury. It may also be too challenging, causing you to lose heart and making it difficult for you to stick with your program. That said, it's likely that you're doing more activity than you're giving yourself credit for, hence the importance of recasting exercise as lifestyle activity. If you doubt that, look back to the table showing calories burned in just ten minutes of activity. It shows that there are many ways to increase your activity level without ever going to a gym, track, or ball field. Remember: *all activity* counts toward creating a healthier lifestyle.

Goal-Setting Worksheet for Getting More Active

Timeline	Plan	Amount of activity
Week 1		
Week 2		
Week 3		
Week 4		
Week 5		
Week 6		
Week 7		
Week 8		

Exercise: Monitoring Your Activity

As with monitoring your diet with a food diary, monitoring your daily lifestyle activities can help you track and understand your patterns around getting active. Therefore, I'm providing a new form, the "Lifestyle Activity Monitoring Form," so you can start tracking this important information. (A downloadable version of this form, which you can use to keep track of your activity level over time, is available at http://www.newharbinger.com/31304; see the back of the book for information on how to access it.) In filling it out, remember that all activity counts. If you do anything active, write it down so you can give yourself credit for doing it. (In chapter 7, I'll discuss rewarding yourself for these types of behaviors.)

Earlier in the chapter, I shared a sample goal-setting worksheet for Bob, with weekly goals for getting more physical activity. As you saw, his plan was very specific and detailed, with concrete goals that can be measured—all important considerations when setting goals. So, as you track your daily activities, you'll want to record what you do with a similar level of detail. After all, the point of having a goal you can measure is to then measure what you actually do. So be sure to get specific when you record your daily activity.

In the followeing pages, I've provided a sample lifestyle activity monitoring form, followed by a blank version for your use.

Sample Lifestyle Activity Monitoring Form

Day	Type of activity	Duration	Notes
Monday	Walking in my neighborhood	20 minutes	It was a pretty, sunny day, and I noticed that I felt a lot happier when I got home.
Tuesday	Walking at the grocery store	15 minutes	I parked at a far corner of the parking lot so I'd have to walk farther.
Tuesday	Sweeping and vacuuming floors	20 minutes	I had to do this anyway, so it's kind of cool that it counts as activity.
Wednesday	Day off		I need to remind myself that it's okay to take a day off. I don't need to increase my activity level every day in the beginning.
Thursday	On a visit to my sister, taking the stairs to the eighth floor to her apartment	20 minutes	I took several breaks and was tired by the time I got to the top, but I felt as though I'd really accomplished something by the time I got to the eighth floor.
Friday	Standing	60 minutes	Instead of sitting during the 30-minute bus ride to and from work, I stood.
Saturday	Playing with my niece	45 minutes	I followed my niece around as she played at my sister's house, including kicking a soccer ball with her for fifteen minutes.
Sunday	Day off		This may be a good day to rest and reflect on what I did over the past week.

Lifestyle Activity Monitoring Form

Day	Type of activity	Duration	Notes

As with food diaries, there are many different options beyond written forms, including smartphone apps and computer programs. If you like that kind of technology, electronic tracking is a perfectly acceptable alternative. Here are some apps that can be helpful for tracking your lifestyle activities:

- **MyFitnessPal.** This online tool, also available as an app, is very popular among my clients who are trying to create a healthier lifestyle. It allows you to record the foods you consume as well as your daily exercise. It also calculates the number of calories burned in the exercise you record.

- **Argus.** Argus is an iPhone app that tracks your activities directly by using the phone's GPS to monitor your movement. So, as long as you have your phone with you and its on, you'll be recording your physical activity. Other features of this app include monitoring your diet, weight, and water consumption. Argus is free, but because it uses the phone's GPS, it will drain your phone's battery fairly quickly.

- **Moves.** This app, which is available for both iPhone and Android, also uses the phone's GPS to record your movements and activity level. It can automatically tell whether you're walking, running, or biking, versus taking public transit or riding in a car. It displays a timeline of your day showing how much time you spent doing different activities. Like Argus, it can also deplete your phone battery fairly quickly.

Some Simple Stretches

Stretching is a great way to increase your lifestyle activity because it can help both your body and your mind. It improves flexibility, keeps muscles loose, helps decrease risk of injury by preparing your muscles for an activity, and supplies blood and nutrients to your muscles, which can help reduce muscle soreness. And if you take big, deep breaths while stretching, it can also calm the mind, provide a mental break, and give your body a chance to recharge. Just five to ten minutes of stretching is enough, so this is an easy thing to add to your daily routine.

Here are a few simple stretches that will help you keep your major muscle groups flexible and healthy.

Standing Toe Touch

1. Stand with your feet shoulder-width apart and knees slightly bent.

2. Slowly bend forward, hinging at your hips and reaching your hands toward your toes. If you can't reach your toes, that's okay. It's important to build flexibility slowly. Just bend forward as far as you comfortably can, then a bit farther, so you feel a slight stretch.

3. Hold the stretch for ten to thirty seconds, making sure you continue to breathe, then slowly return to a standing posture.

4. Repeat the stretch two more times, trying to reach a bit farther each time.

Quadriceps Stretch

1. Stand near a chair or wall with your legs together.

2. Bend one knee, raising your foot behind you, and grab that foot with the hand on the same side. To maintain your balance, stretch the opposite arm out forward or hold on to the chair or wall.

3. Bring your heel as close to your buttock as you comfortably can, then bring it just a bit closer, so you feel a gentle stretch.

4. Hold the stretch for ten to thirty seconds, making sure you continue to breathe. Slowly release and return to the starting position.

5. Do the stretch on the other side, then repeat two more times on each side.

Side Bends

1. Stand with your feet shoulder-width apart and your back straight, then stretch both arms up over your head and clasp your hands together.

2. Gently bend to the right as far as you comfortably can, then go just a bit farther, until you feel a gentle stretch.

3. Hold for ten to thirty seconds, making sure you continue to breathe. Slowly return to the starting position.

4. Do the stretch on the other side, then repeat two more times on each side, trying to stretch a bit farther each time.

Triceps Stretch

1. Stand with your feet shoulder-width apart and your back straight. Stretch your right arm over your head, then bend it at the elbow to bring your right hand toward your mid-back.

2. Raise your left arm alongside your head, bend it at the elbow, and grasp your right elbow with your left hand. Gently pull your right elbow downward and back.

3. Hold the stretch for ten to thirty seconds, then gently release.

4. Do the stretch on the other side, then repeat two more times on each side.

Summary

- People with bipolar disorder are at greater risk for developing cardiovascular disease than the general population.

- Exercise can benefit your mental health (for example, helping with sleep, anxiety, or depression) and physical health (for example, reducing risk of diabetes or stroke). It isn't clear, however, whether exercise helps manage mania.

- Consider renaming "exercise" as "lifestyle activity" to reflect that there are many ways to burn calories and lead a healthier, more active life.

- For healthy adults, 150 minutes of moderate-intensity aerobic lifestyle activity per week is recommended.

- Strength training and stretching are also important for health and wellness.

- Start a new activity program slowly, setting specific, realistic goals and increasing your activity level gradually.

- Track your daily lifestyle activity.

Chapter 6

Changing How You
Think About Exercise

Many people have trouble exercising on a regular basis, such as four or five days per week. In fact, the National Center for Health Statistics (2013) recently did a large survey and found that 50 percent of people weren't engaging in aerobic exercise regularly. Strength training was even less popular, with only one of out every four people meeting recommended guidelines. Unfortunately, people with bipolar disorder tend to exercise even less frequently than others. One large study found that 71 percent of people with bipolar disorder reported exercising less than three times per week, compared to 66 percent for the general population (Kilbourne et al. 2007).

So, given the many benefits of exercise (some of them discussed in chapter 5), why do people have so much trouble exercising? There seem to be two major obstacles:

- The ways people think about exercise

- What people choose to do instead of exercising

In this chapter, we'll tackle the first obstacle: thoughts about exercise. In chapter 7, we'll work on the second obstacle and how you can use rewards to overcome behaviors that get in the way of exercising. Specifically, we'll take a look at how to reward behaviors that support creating a healthy lifestyle in order to make it more likely that you'll choose healthy behaviors in the future.

Assumptions About Exercise

Many people's first encounter with exercise is during childhood, in organized sports such as baseball, basketball, track and field, and soccer. These types of sports are high-intensity forms of exercise, requiring a lot of physical effort. As a result, people tend to assume that exercising means doing a lot of physical work. No wonder people think exercising is hard!

Although it would be great to be doing such high-intensity activities as an adult, for people who haven't been active in a long time, it can seem overwhelming to start a new exercise program by doing such high-intensity activities, especially sports they haven't played in ten, fifteen, or twenty years. This is one reason why I advocate renaming "exercise" as "lifestyle activity," as discussed in chapter 5. The name "lifestyle activity" highlights that there are many different ways to exercise and that low-intensity activities, such as walking downstairs or light gardening, still count as exercise. They give you many ways of burning calories and becoming healthier by reducing cholesterol levels and decreasing blood pressure.

Take a moment to consider what assumptions you have about exercising. I discussed false assumptions in chapter 4, but as a reminder, assumptions are thoughts you believe to be true that may not actually be true, or consistent with reality. They are guesses or theories, not facts, though they may contain a grain of truth. For example, the thought that exercise is very difficult is an assumption; it isn't necessarily true. If you make a point of engaging in short periods of low-intensity exercise as you begin a new activity program, it probably won't feel very hard, and it will certainly feel much easier than if you suddenly start engaging in long bouts of high-intensity exercise.

Also, be aware that people with bipolar disorder tend to make more false assumptions when either depressed or manic. As discussed in previous chapters, these mood episodes distort your thinking, and this makes it difficult to have objective, factual thoughts, especially about yourself. Consider the following example.

> Emily struggled with her mood for several years, but she didn't see a doctor until she became very depressed at age forty-two. Emily's doctor diagnosed her with bipolar II disorder based on her brief but distinct episodes of elevated mood and her many episodes of major depression. Her doctor prescribed a mood-stabilizing medication and also recommended that Emily start exercising more often to manage her depression.
>
> Emily felt doubtful about exercising. Her impression was that she hadn't exercised in over fifteen years. She enjoyed horseback riding, gardening, and doing

major chores around her house, such as cleaning out her attic, but she thought she wasn't ready to start exercising. She felt sad about this. She wanted to exercise and knew it would be good for her. But she just couldn't picture herself doing the sports she'd enjoyed as a teen, such as swimming and playing basketball. And it seemed even more unrealistic to her that she could start doing these sports now that she'd been diagnosed with bipolar disorder and had to take medication. So she filled the prescription and started taking the medication, but she didn't make any changes in her physical activity.

Exercise: Identifying Emily's Assumptions

What assumptions is Emily making? Below, I've listed some of the thoughts Emily had after leaving her doctor's office. To give you some practice in distinguishing between facts (things that are true) and assumptions (theories or guesses), read through the list below. Circle "Fact" if Emily's thought seems to be true, and "Assumption" if the thought seems to be a theory or guess.

1. *I have bipolar disorder.*   Fact   Assumption

2. *I'll always be depressed.*   Fact   Assumption

3. *Exercise can help me manage my depression.*   Fact   Assumption

4. *I have to exercise.*   Fact   Assumption

5. *Bipolar medications cause weight gain.*   Fact   Assumption

6. *Having bipolar disorder makes it more difficult to exercise.*   Fact   Assumption

7. *I haven't exercised in fifteen years.*   Fact   Assumption

8. *I haven't gone swimming or played basketball in fifteen years.*   Fact   Assumption

9. *I don't know how to exercise.*   Fact   Assumption

10. *I'll never be able to exercise again.*   Fact   Assumption

Answers: 1. Fact; 2. Assumption; 3. Fact; 4. Assumption; 5. Assumption; 6. Assumption; 7. Assumption; 8. Fact; 9. Fact; 10. Assumption

The truth is, only three of those statements are facts: 1, 3, and 8. But if you thought the other statements were facts, you are not alone. Among people with bipolar disorder, these are very common assumptions. Remember, assumptions may have a grain of truth. So, although having bipolar disorder may mean that *at times* it's more difficult to exercise than it is for other people, this isn't always true. After all, there are many people with bipolar disorder who exercise more regularly than others who don't have bipolar disorder. It's also worth noting that statement 7 is an assumption—Emily must have done some type of exercise, or lifestyle activity in fifteen years.

Identifying Your Own Assumptions About Exercise

To identify your own assumptions about exercise, you first need to identify your thoughts about exercise. In chapter 4, you learned how to identify your automatic thoughts. Now I'll help you identify your automatic thoughts about exercise—all of the thoughts that just come to mind on this topic. This requires a bit of soul-searching and being very honest with yourself about what you think. For example, Emily may have found it difficult to write down her thought that she'll never exercise again, but this is obviously a key thought for Emily to overcome in order to start making lifestyle changes.

I've also heard people say that they don't know how to start an exercise program, that they believe exercise is too overwhelming, or that they simply don't see themselves ever exercising again. These are all important and very limiting automatic thoughts about exercise, so it's important to examine them carefully to determine whether they're facts or assumptions.

In chapter 4, I provided some guidance on identifying automatic thoughts. But because this can be tricky, let's go through a similar process here to strengthen your ability to identify automatic thoughts. To provide some context, let's consider another example.

John has bipolar disorder. He's lived alone since moving out of his parents' house five years ago. He works full-time and finds his job very challenging. It's hard for him to manage his irritability toward his coworkers when he's depressed. He also has difficulty getting to work on time. A friend recently suggested that John start exercising as a way to improve his depression, but John believes he's too busy and doesn't have time to exercise.

To identify what some of John's automatic thoughts about exercise might be, let's use those same key questions outlined in chapter 4. I've provided potential automatic thoughts below; you might have ideas about others.

What went through my mind just as I thought about exercising? *Exercise won't help me.*

What do these thoughts mean about me? *I don't think that anything will help my depression.*

What do these thoughts mean about me in the big picture (for my life and my future)? *I won't be able to manage my depression.*

What do I fear might happen if these thoughts are true? *If exercise won't help me, maybe nothing will, and I'm afraid that might lead to losing my job.*

What's the worst thing that could happen if these thoughts are true? *I'll get very depressed and lose my job and then my house.*

What do these thoughts suggest in terms of what other people might think or feel about me? *People will think I'm a loser because I'll be overweight, alone, and not have a house or a job.*

What do these thoughts mean about other people in general? *Other people are better than me, and they'll think I'm worthless.*

Now that we've identified John's automatic thoughts, the next step is to determine which of them are facts and which are assumptions. You can probably see that many of these thoughts are assumptions. For example, do you think that exercise could help John? And if exercise doesn't improve his depression substantially, could other things help him manage his depression? I hope you're saying "Yes!" to these questions. If you are, then you know that these automatic thoughts can't always be true. They're assumptions.

Likewise, depression and difficulties with coworkers don't necessarily mean that John will lose his job. And even if John were to lose his job, there's a good chance he could find another job. It isn't a given that he'll lose his job or his house. It also isn't a given that he'll end up overweight. All of those are possible future outcomes, but they're just that: possibilities, not facts.

Additionally, many people experience depression, are overweight, don't own homes, or are unemployed while still being very worthy. Perhaps you know someone who's currently unemployed but still volunteers at a church, local food pantry, or another charitable organization. Maybe you have friends or family members who are overweight but very hardworking and kind. You may also know people who are depressed and therefore more irritable and have difficulty getting motivated to do things. Of course, they're still worthy people. The goal here is to see that thoughts aren't always true or factual, and that the worst-case scenario is typically unlikely.

Exercise: Identifying Your Automatic Thoughts and Assumptions About Exercise

Now it's time for you to identify your own automatic thoughts about exercise, and then to determine whether they're facts or assumptions. To help you do this, take a moment to imagine that you're just about to do some sort of physical activity. For example, maybe you're trying to think of what exercise you could do this week. Stop right there and notice what's going through your mind. You may want to use the same helpful questions to identify your automatic thoughts about exercise:

What went through my mind just as I thought about exercising?

What do these thoughts about exercise mean about me?

What do these thoughts mean about me in the big picture (for my life and my future)?

What do I fear might happen if these thoughts are true?

What's the worst thing that could happen if these thoughts are true?

What do these thoughts suggest in terms of what other people might think or feel about me?

What do these thoughts mean about other people in general?

As you identify automatic thoughts, write them in the worksheet that follows. Once you've completed your list, go back and, for each thought, circle "Fact" if you think that thought is always true, or "Assumption" if it's a theory, a guess, or not always true.

My Automatic Thoughts About Exercise

	Fact	Assumption
	Fact	Assumption
	Fact	Assumption
	Fact	Assumption
	Fact	Assumption
	Fact	Assumption
	Fact	Assumption
	Fact	Assumption
	Fact	Assumption
	Fact	Assumption
	Fact	Assumption

What did you discover in doing this exercise? Do you have some assumptions about exercise that may be getting in the way of increasing your activity level? If you do, you are not alone. This is very common. Fortunately, these thoughts do not need to be obstacles to exercising. You can challenge them and ultimately overcome them. The next exercise will help you do just that.

Challenging Your Assumptions About Exercise

People generally know that increasing their activity level is important for health and wellness, yet many still don't do it. Why? Often assumptions are involved. The mind uses assumptions as excuses for not getting more active. Below are some assumptions people commonly have about increasing their activity level and some examples of evidence against them.

Assumption: I don't have enough time to exercise more.

Evidence against this thought: *Ten minutes of increased lifestyle activity, such as walking upstairs, can count as exercise. I also seem to find time to do other things, such as watching TV, so I can find twenty to thirty minutes a day to increase my lifestyle activity if I choose to make it a priority.*

Assumption: I have too many other things to cope with that are more important than exercise.

Evidence against this thought: *Increasing my lifestyle activity can help me in two very important ways, improving both my physical health and my bipolar disorder. Becoming more active has helped many other people become more healthy by lowering their blood pressure and cholesterol levels and losing weight. This is particularly important for me since my bipolar disorder puts me at increased risk for these health issues. Research also shows that being more active can help with depression and ease the symptoms of bipolar disorder.*

Assumption: I'm too tired to exercise.

Evidence against this thought: *I'll probably feel tired often; this is a symptom of depression. If I really want to increase my lifestyle activity and be healthier, I'll always need to fight through this feeling. To do this, I can increase my activity level by doing more of the things I already enjoy* *doing, like playing with my niece or walking my dog. I can also remind myself that I generally feel better when I'm more active.*

Assumption: I don't know how to exercise or what to do.

Evidence against this thought: *Increasing my activity level can involve anything that gets me moving; it doesn't have to be an intense or complicated activity, such as an organized sport. I can start by doing more of any physical activity that I'm already doing. I can also seek support from friends who enjoy being active.*

Assumption: My weight or health is hopeless, and exercising more won't help.

Evidence against this thought: *Studies have shown that losing just 7 percent of my current body weight can substantially improve my overall physical health. For me, that would be about fourteen pounds. If I lose one pound per week for fourteen weeks, I'll lose fourteen pounds and hit this goal in less than four months! I could even lose just half a pound per week for twenty-eight weeks. It would take longer, but I'd still achieve this goal.*

Assumption: Exercise is boring.

Evidence against this thought: *Given that any increase in activity can qualify as exercise, it can't be boring. I need to focus on physical activities I enjoy, such as walking in the mall or dancing. I can also make activities more interesting by listening to music or doing them with a friend. For activities like riding a stationary bike, I could even read a book or watch a show or movie.*

Assumption: Exercising won't help me. I've tried it before and it didn't help.

Evidence against this thought: *I may not have kept it up long enough or increased my activity level enough to see any benefits. I also may have been so depressed that I didn't recognize how it helped me. In fact, my friends have told me that I seemed to have more energy and focus when I was more active.*

Assumption: I'm too overweight now to exercise.

Evidence against this thought: *Anyone can increase their activity level; I just need to start off slowly. For example, maybe I could start by watching the first part of my TV show standing up instead of sitting. I could also go to the park twice a week instead of once a week to walk around more.*

Changing Your Assumptions About Exercise

After identifying assumptions that serve as obstacles to exercise and examining the evidence against these thoughts, the next step is to work on changing these thoughts. As you'll recall from chapter 4, this is called cognitive restructuring. Before reading on, you may want to review the work you did in chapter 4 on changing your thoughts about your diet. Sometimes this is as simple as changing the words you use, which is why I advocate relabeling "exercise" as "lifestyle activity." Of course, if you find that another term works better for you, then that's the one to use. The main point is, which sounds more appealing—"exercising more" or "going for a walk and enjoying some sunshine and fresh air"? Likewise, which sounds more achievable—"dieting" or "eating reasonable amounts of food"?

Exercise: Assessing the Believability of Alternative Thoughts

The previous section covered some common assumptions about exercising more and provided some evidence against them. Now it's your turn to work on changing your assumptions about increasing your activity level. Turn back to the exercise "Identifying Your Automatic Thoughts and Assumptions About Exercise" and, for all thoughts you labeled as assumptions, write them in the left-hand column ("Assumptions") in the worksheet provided. Then look for evidence against these assumptions and use that evidence to come up with new, alternative thoughts that will support you in making healthy changes. Write your new, alternative thoughts in the middle column ("Alternative thoughts"). In the right-hand column, rate how much you believe each new thought using a scale of 0 to 100 percent, with 100 percent meaning you completely believe the new thought and 0 meaning you don't believe the new thought at all.

Assumptions	Alternative thoughts	Believe? (0–100%)

If you find that your believability rating for any new thought is less than 50 percent, you are not alone. As discussed in chapter 4 in the beginning it can be difficult to believe new thoughts. To believe them more strongly, we need to practice them.

Using Coping Cards to Practice Alternative Thoughts

Practicing your new, alternative thoughts about increasing your lifestyle activity requires having these thoughts easily available to you. As discussed in chapter 4, coping cards are one way to practice alternative thoughts, and there are various ways to set them up. In chapter 4, you created cards that each had a new thought on one side and strategies for enacting that new approach on the other side.

Another way to set these cards up is to write an old assumption on one side of each card and your new, alternative thought on the other side. If you like, you can also include some of the evidence supporting the new thought. This is essentially a way to take the work that you did in the previous exercise with you as you go about your day. Then, anytime you find yourself caught up in one of your old assumptions, you can refer to the card for that assumption to remind yourself of your new thought.

As mentioned in chapter 4, it's fine to use the notes app on your phone or to set up reminders to pop up on your phone rather than using index cards. Other ways to make your new thoughts more a part of your life include e-mailing them to yourself or posting reminders around your house, in your car, or at your workplace.

The exact strategy you use doesn't matter; the goal is to read or say these new, alternative thoughts several times every day and take some time to think them and think about them. If you just mindlessly read them, that won't help. Your brain won't automatically switch over to thinking new thoughts; you need to engage in an active process of training your brain to think alternative thoughts, and you need to actively practice them every day.

When Alternative Thoughts Aren't Enough

If you try practicing new, alternative thoughts for about a month and continue to have negative assumptions about increasing your activity level, you may need to strengthen the evidence in favor of these thoughts or generate new alternative thoughts. Here are a few tips that may help:

- Revisit any assumptions you're having difficulty changing and try to come up with some new evidence against them.

- Generate different alternative thoughts. To find more effective alternatives, identify positive thoughts you use to help you do other things, such as cleaning your house, getting up in the morning, or being nice to an annoying boss.

- Imagine that your assumptions about increasing your activity level are someone else's assumptions. Try to persuade this imaginary person to engage in more activity. What would you say to convince someone to do more physical activity? Write these thoughts down and try them for yourself.

- Show your assumptions to friends or family members and ask them to challenge the assumptions. They may be able to provide more compelling evidence or alternative thoughts that will be more effective.

If you continue to struggle with changing your assumptions, you may want to take a break from focusing on your thinking and start working on changing your behaviors. Chapter 7 will help you do just that. You may also want to revisit the discussion of the preparation and action stages of change, in chapter 1.

Summary

- Many people have difficulty exercising.

- One reason people have trouble exercising is that they have negative automatic thoughts and assumptions about exercise.

- Changing your ideas about exercise can be as simple as giving it a new name, such as "lifestyle activity."

- Changing your assumptions about increasing your activity level is a four-step process:

  1. Identify your automatic thoughts about exercise.

  2. Determine which automatic thoughts are assumptions.

  3. Find the evidence against these assumptions and use it to create new, alternative thoughts.

  4. Practice your new, alternative thoughts.

Chapter 7

Learning to Reward Yourself

I want to start this chapter with a bold idea: you deserve to reward yourself. This is an especially challenging idea for most people who have bipolar disorder. However, rewarding yourself can help you make positive changes to your lifestyle. So, in this chapter, I'll help you identify rewards that will work for you and provide motivation to make important changes in your life.

People with Bipolar Disorder Don't Often Reward Themselves

One symptom of depression is having a sense of worthlessness. If you've experienced depression, you may sometimes believe that you're worthless. This belief often causes people to think they are doing things wrong, should be doing more, or are fundamentally flawed in some way. When people are depressed, their thoughts become overly negative, to the point that they are often inaccurate or distorted. Therefore, it isn't unusual for people who are depressed to not notice when they do things well or accomplish things that are difficult. As a result, they seldom believe that they deserve to be rewarded.

This is a problem. If you don't reward yourself, how can you acknowledge that you've done something well? And if you're unable to recognize that you've done something well, you'll just keep thinking you're worthless, so the cycle continues. You need to break this vicious cycle; otherwise it will just keep going around and around, never ending.

The Importance of Rewards

Rewards are an effective tool for breaking this vicious cycle. If you stop to reward yourself, you ensure that you see you've done something right. And after all, everyone does *something* right. Let's consider an example.

Sue has been depressed for several months, but her depression deepened recently when her elderly aunt got sick. Sue feels responsible for watching over her aunt and taking care of her, and tries to visit her several times each month. But her aunt lives across the state—over five hours away by car. So Sue is driving long distances at least four times per month. These long drives are emotionally painful for Sue because she spends much of the time focusing on her negative thoughts. To help with that problem, she listens to audiobooks to distract herself from her thoughts.

Sue is overweight, and before her aunt got sick, she'd been working on eating better and being more active, which had helped her lose some weight. But now she's stopped losing weight because she doesn't tend to cook when she has to travel a lot. Plus, she's been exercising less because her routine has been disrupted. Still, she's tried to be thoughtful about the foods she selects at restaurants, and she takes the stairs at the nursing home where her aunt lives.

Overall, Sue's life has become more stressful. She's worried about her aunt's health, and she's taken on the responsibilities of managing her aunt's finances and health care and the sale of her home. Sue's also almost completely stopped doing things that typically make her feel better, like reading, watching movies, and visiting with friends. She's started drinking more, and she's fallen back on an old habit of overspending, going on a few shopping sprees that she couldn't really afford. She's become overwhelmed, and her struggles with her weight and fitness, combined with the challenges she faces in taking care of her aunt's affairs, have led Sue to believe that she can't do anything right. She feels very alone and sad.

Given Sue's situation, do you think she's likely to reward herself? It seems doubtful that she will, given that she believes she can't do anything right. But is that an accurate belief? Or is Sue doing anything she deserves to be rewarded for? (I hope your answer to that second question is "Yes!")

Take a moment now to reread Sue's story and identify things she's doing right. Here are some of the things I notice.

- **Visiting her aunt.** Sue is keeping her aunt company and showing her that she cares about her.

- **Listening to audiobooks while driving.** This is a skill Sue is using to distract herself from her negative thoughts.

- **Trying to choose healthy options at restaurants.** This will improve Sue's nutrition and help her manage her weight.

- **Using the stairs rather than the elevator.** This increases Sue's activity level.

- **Managing her aunt's finances.** This helps her aunt and may reduce her aunt's stress.

- **Selling her aunt's house.** This is a tremendous amount of work. This could be important for her aunt's finances, and her aunt probably isn't able to take on the task.

- **Overseeing her aunt's health care.** Again, this is a great help to her aunt.

- **Maintaining her weight.** Although Sue isn't losing weight, she's been able to maintain her current weight during this stressful time.

All of these behaviors are worth rewarding. It's important for Sue to learn to see this. As it is, she may believe that these are all duties or things she *should* be doing, and therefore not worthy of rewards. In fact, she may tend to focus only on the minor difficulties that she has in performing these tasks, such as occasionally taking the elevator or making minor errors when handling her aunt's bills. Or she may focus solely on things she isn't doing that she thinks she should, like exercising and losing weight.

Does any of this sound familiar? Have you had similar thoughts? Like Sue, you may focus excessively on the negative, not seeing all the things you're doing right. Hopefully the previous chapters have made it clear that people's thoughts about things aren't always accurate. So if you believe that you've done nothing today that deserves a reward, be sure to check the accuracy of your thinking. Everyone does something each day that's worth acknowledging with a reward.

A Potential Problem with Rewards

At this point, there may be a few folks reading this book who are saying, "You're right! I should be rewarding myself more frequently. Now I have a reason to eat my favorite dessert, drink a glass of wine, or skip exercising today. Those will be my rewards!" You can probably see how this could be problematic. A reward should appropriately match the *target behavior*, meaning the behavior that you're rewarding. In addition, rewards shouldn't feed into problem behaviors, such as overeating, substance abuse, excessive spending, or skipping exercise.

To illustrate rewards that don't appropriately match the target behavior, let's revisit Sue's example. Here are some inappropriate rewards for Sue's target behaviors, along with explanations of why these rewards are problematic.

Target behavior: Visiting her aunt

Example of inappropriate reward: Buying herself a new car

Why inappropriate: This feeds into Sue's overspending problem.

Target behavior: Listening to audiobooks while driving

Example of inappropriate reward: Eating dessert every night

Why inappropriate: This furthers Sue's overeating problem.

Target behavior: Trying to choose healthy food options at restaurants

Example of inappropriate reward: Having a glass of wine at each meal

Why inappropriate: This contributes to Sue's drinking problem.

Target behavior: Using the stairs rather than the elevator

Example of inappropriate reward: Not exercising for the rest of the week

Why inappropriate: This feeds into Sue's difficulty in exercising.

Target behavior: Helping her aunt with her finances

Example of inappropriate reward: Ignoring her own bills

Why inappropriate: Sue isn't taking care of herself.

Target behavior: Selling her aunt's home

Example of inappropriate reward: Giving herself some of the money from the sale without her aunt's approval

Why inappropriate: This is unfair to her aunt, which is contrary to Sue's goal of helping her aunt.

Target behavior: Managing her aunt's health care

Example of inappropriate reward: Not going to her own support groups and medical appointments

Why inappropriate: Sue isn't taking care of herself.

Target behavior: Not gaining weight

Example of inappropriate reward: Going on a shopping spree for new clothes that exceeds her budget

Why inappropriate: This contributes to Sue's overspending problem.

As you can see, rewards can be problematic if they don't match the target behavior well or if they feed into problem behaviors. Given that bipolar disorder makes it more difficult to think accurately at times, it's very important that you make a point of identifying in advance rewards that will work well for you. The next exercise will help you do just that.

Exercise: Identifying Appropriate Rewards

To help you identify rewards that could be appropriate for you, consider this question: What are some activities you enjoy doing? Give it some thought and make a list of what you come up with.

1. _____

2. _____

3. _____

4. _____

5. _____

6. _____

7. _____

8. _____

9. _____

10. _____

If you have bipolar disorder, and particularly if you're depressed right now, you may have trouble identifying enjoyable activities. To help you brainstorm some ideas, read through the following list of positive activities (adapted with permission from McKay, Wood, and Brantley 2007). Circle any activities that you'd like to try or that you're currently doing and would like to increase.

Positive Activities

Talk to a friend on the telephone.

Go out and visit a friend.

Invite a friend to come to your home.

Text-message your friends.

Organize a party.

Exercise.

Lift weights.

Do yoga, tai chi, or Pilates, or take classes to learn.

Stretch your muscles.

Go for a long walk in a park or someplace else that's peaceful.

Go outside and watch the clouds.

Go jog.

Ride your bike.

Go for a swim.

Go hiking.

Do something exciting, like surfing, rock climbing, skiing, skydiving, motorcycle riding, or kayaking, or go learn how to do one of these things.

Go to your local playground and join a game being played or watch a game.

Go play something you can do by yourself if no one else is around,

like basketball, bowling, handball, miniature golf, billiards, or hitting a tennis ball against the wall.

Get a massage; this can also help soothe your emotions.

Get out of your house, even if you just sit outside.

Go for a drive in your car or go for a ride on public transportation.

Plan a trip to a place you've never been before.

Sleep or take a nap.

Cook your favorite dish or meal.

Cook a recipe that you've never tried before.

Take a cooking class.

Go outside and play with your pet.

Go borrow a friend's dog and take it to the park.

Give your pet a bath.

Go outside and watch the birds and other animals.

Find something funny to do, like reading the Sunday comics.

Watch a funny movie (start collecting funny movies to watch when you're feeling overwhelmed with pain).

Go to the movie theater and watch whatever's playing.

Watch television.

Listen to the radio.

Go to a sporting event, like a baseball or football game.

Play a game with a friend.

Play solitaire.

Play video games.

Go online to chat.

Visit your favorite websites.

Create your own website.

Create your own blog.

Join an Internet dating service.

Sell something you don't want on the Internet.

Buy something on the Internet.

Do a puzzle with a lot of pieces.

Go shopping.

Go get a haircut.

Go to a spa.

Go to a library.

Go to a bookstore and read.

Go to your favorite café for coffee or tea.

Visit a museum or local art gallery.

Go to the mall or the park and watch other people; try to imagine what they're thinking.

Pray or meditate.

Go to your church, synagogue, temple, or other place of worship.

Join a group at your place of worship.

Write a letter to God.

Call a family member you haven't spoken to in a long time.

Learn a new language.

Sing or learn how to sing.

Play a musical instrument or learn how to play one.

Write a song.

Listen to some upbeat, happy music (start collecting happy songs for times when you're feeling overwhelmed).

Turn on some loud music and dance in your room.

Memorize lines from your favorite movie, play, or song.

Make a movie or video with your camcorder.

Take photographs.

Join a public speaking group and write a speech.

Participate in a local theater group.

Sing in a local choir.

Join a club.

Plant a garden.

Work outside.

Knit, crochet, or sew—or learn how to.

Make a scrapbook with pictures.

Paint your nails.

Change your hair color.

Take a bubble bath or shower.

Work on your car, truck, motorcycle, or bicycle.

Sign up for a class that excites you at a local college, adult school, or online.

Read your favorite book, magazine, paper, or poem.

Read a trashy celebrity magazine.

Write a letter to a friend or family member.

Write things you like about yourself on a picture of your body or draw them on a photograph of yourself.

Write a poem, story, movie, or play about your life or someone else's life.

Write in your journal or diary about what happened to you today.

Write a loving letter to yourself when you're feeling good and keep it with you to read when you're feeling upset.

Make a list of ten things you're good at or that you like about yourself when you're feeling good and keep it with you to read when you're feeling upset.

Draw a picture.

Paint a picture with a brush or your fingers.

Masturbate.

Have sex with someone you care about.

Make a list of the people you admire and want to be like—it can be anyone real or fictional throughout history. Describe what you admire about these people.

Write a story about the craziest, funniest, or sexiest thing that has ever happened to you.

Make a list of ten things you would like to do before you die.

Make a list of ten celebrities you would like to be friends with and describe why.

Make a list of ten celebrities you would like to have sex with and describe why.

Write a letter to someone who has made your life better and tell that person why your life is better. (You don't have to send the letter if you don't want to.)

Create your own list of pleasurable activities.

Once you've listed at least ten activities that you enjoy doing, consider whether any of these activities feed into unhealthy behaviors that you're trying to stop. Look at each activity separately and ask yourself whether it supports unhealthy behaviors or has the potential to be problematic for you. Examples of unhealthy behaviors include drinking, substance abuse, overspending, eating unhealthy foods or overeating, doing less physical activity, or isolating yourself from others. With that in mind, go through your list and cross out any activities that are inappropriate rewards.

Taking a Closer Look at Appropriate Rewards

To help you with any difficulties in identifying enjoyable activities or ruling out those that are inappropriate, let's consider another example.

Sharon, who has bipolar disorder, is overweight and often experiences depression. As a result, she struggles to feel interested in things. She lacks motivation and energy and often feels tired, irritable, and sad. A typical day for Sharon involves staying in bed until almost noon, watching TV on the couch, drinking a six-pack of beer, not showering, and buying things she doesn't need online.

At a friend's recommendation, Sharon decided to try rewarding herself with positive activities. To that end, she created the following list:

- *Sleep until 1 p.m.*

- *Get a pedicure.*

- *Watch television.*

- *Rest on the couch.*

- *Stay inside.*

- *Take a hot bath.*

- *Sit on the back porch.*

- *Surf the web.*

- *Drink a beer.*

- *Call a friend.*

- *Buy gifts for neighbors.*

- *Eat a favorite dessert.*

What do you think of Sharon's list? Should she use all of these activities as rewards, or do some of them perhaps encourage unhealthy behaviors? Review Sharon's list and circle any activities that seem as though they could potentially be problematic for her.

Now let's go through that list item by item. Below, I've detailed whether each activity is an appropriate reward and why it's appropriate or inappropriate. For those that might be problematic, the right-hand column provides examples of how Sharon could modify the activity to create a more appropriate reward.

Activity	Appropriate?	Why or why not?	Revised reward
Sleep until 1 p.m.	No	Sharon seems to spend too much time in bed. She needs to encourage herself to get out of bed.	Take a short afternoon nap on days when she gets out of bed by 9 a.m.
Get a pedicure.	Yes	This isn't too costly and Sharon currently isn't doing this regularly.	
Watch television.	No	Sharon is already watching a lot of television. She needs to encourage herself to watch less television.	Watch one favorite show per day or a special movie three days per week.
Rest on the couch.	No	Sharon is already spending a lot of time on the couch. She needs to encourage herself to get off the couch. She also needs to decrease her isolation.	Invite a friend over and rest in a comfortable chair while they visit.
Stay inside.	No	Sharon spends a lot of time inside and needs to encourage herself to go outside.	After running an errand or going for a walk, rest inside for one hour.

Activity	Appropriate?	Why or why not?	Revised reward
Take a hot bath.	Yes	This is an enjoyable activity that doesn't feed into any unhealthy behaviors, and it also supports better self-care.	
Sit on the back porch.	Yes	This supports the healthy behavior of getting out of the house more, so it's a great reward.	
Surf the web.	No	Sharon is spending too much money on the web, and this could feed into that unhealthy behavior.	Spend one hour on the web per day—without buying anything.
Drink a beer.	No	This feeds into Sharon's unhealthy behavior of drinking too much.	Have another favorite beverage, such as tea or coffee.
Call a friend.	Yes	This is a great reward because it decreases Sharon's isolation and also helps maintain her social support.	
Buy gifts for neighbors.	No	This feeds into Sharon's overspending problem.	Write cards to her neighbors or buy an inexpensive gift for one friend.
Eat a favorite dessert.	No	Sharon is overweight and needs to be very careful about how she uses food as a reward.	Have a small amount of her favorite dessert on days when she exercises for more than thirty minutes.

Did you identify the same activities in Sharon's list as potentially being problematic? If not, that's okay. We can't really know what might be problematic without talking to Sharon. The main point is to recognize that not all enjoyable activities are positive or healthy. Given that you have bipolar disorder, you may have trouble accurately determining which activities are positive and which aren't, just like Sharon. Having bipolar disorder can make it more challenging to choose good rewards because, when you're depressed or manic, you may not be able to see the situation clearly. You may also tend to be more impulsive than people who don't have bipolar disorder, which can make it more difficult to carefully choose rewards. So, as you get started on choosing rewards for yourself, I encourage you to work with a friend, family member, or other support person to help you determine which rewards are appropriate for you.

Putting It All Together: The Rewards Chart

At this point, I hope that I've convinced you of two things. First, it's important to reward yourself. Everyone deserves a reward. Second, inappropriate rewards can be problematic, so you need to choose your rewards carefully. There's one final important point in regard to rewards. It's best to match them with target behaviors—the goals you're aiming toward—because rewards provide motivation to do things. A helpful strategy for matching rewards with target behaviors is to create a rewards chart, setting forth realistic, measurable target behaviors (goals) and specifying the reward for accomplishing each. To see how it works, let's consider another example.

Bill, a college student recently diagnosed with bipolar disorder, is majoring in studio arts. He's finishing up his sophomore year and looking forward to going home for the summer to spend more time with his family and to work at a youth camp with his friends. Since his diagnosis, Bill has been working on creating a healthier lifestyle to manage his bipolar disorder, with a focus on maintaining his sobriety, keeping a regular schedule, eating more nutritiously, exercising, and spending less time isolated in his room. He'd like to continue to improve his lifestyle over the summer, but he's worried because his friends and family don't share his enthusiasm for these kinds of positive changes. For example, his family drinks a lot of alcohol, and many of his friends and family members don't eat well or exercise regularly.

One way Bill can stick to his plan to live a healthier lifestyle while he's back home is to create a rewards chart. First, he needs to identify target behaviors, keeping them specific and realistic. In keeping with the guidelines on goal setting in chapter 2, I've designed the rewards chart to list a main goal in the left-hand column. For his goals, Bill might choose maintaining a regular schedule, staying sober, eating more nutritious foods, isolating himself less, and exercising regularly. The middle column of the rewards chart has space to list very specific target behaviors that align with the goal that follows. If you review the sample worksheet, you'll see some very specific, achievable target behaviors that Bill has identified as worthy of rewards.

The next step is to identify appropriate rewards that support the target behaviors or at least don't feed problem behaviors. For example, Bill seems particularly worried about maintaining his sobriety while around his friends and family. His bipolar disorder could make this especially challenging, since mood episodes can increase cravings to drink. Therefore, this target behavior should have a substantial reward. Of course, buying a new car or taking a trip to Europe wouldn't be appropriate for just one week of sobriety. However, Bill might decide to reward himself with something very meaningful to him but less expensive, such as buying new art supplies. As a studio arts major, he very much wants these, so spending fifty dollars on new supplies could be very motivating for him. In contrast, Bill may anticipate that being at home will actually help him maintain a regular schedule because he'll get up when his family members do and eat meals with them. Since this target behavior will be less demanding, the rewards are more modest: sleeping in one morning or doing something relaxing for thirty minutes.

Bill's Rewards Chart

Main goals	Specific target behaviors	Rewards
Maintain a regular schedule (getting up at 9 a.m. and having breakfast at 10 a.m., lunch at 2 p.m., and dinner at 8 p.m.).	If I eat all three meals at the planned times this week	Sleep in one day this week.
	If I get up on time four days this week	Schedule thirty minutes for a relaxing activity, such as reading, taking a long bath, or getting a massage.
Maintain my sobriety.	If I go the entire week without drinking or using marijuana	Buy new art supplies (about $50) for my next studio arts project.
	If I attend at least two AA meetings this week	Watch a favorite show or go to the movies.
Eat more nutritious foods.	If I eat two servings of fruit daily for three days	Have a favorite meal or dessert that's less nutritious, maybe pancakes for dinner.
	If I eat three servings of vegetables daily for three days	Visit a favorite place, such as the beach, a park, a friend's house, or an arcade.
Isolate less.	If I leave the house at least every other day to do something social	Go out for dinner one night at my favorite restaurant.
Exercise regularly.	If I exercise four days this week for at least thirty minutes each time	Buy a small treat for myself, such as a new shirt under $25 or a one-year subscription to my favorite magazine.

Exercise: Creating Your Own Rewards Chart

Now it's time for you to list your own goals, target behaviors, and rewards. A blank worksheet for this purpose is provided; a downloadable version is also available, for rewards charts you might want to create in the future, at http://www.newharbinger.com/31304. See the back of the book for more information.

As you fill out the worksheet, if you have trouble identifying healthy goals that you're excited about achieving, seek support from a friend or family member. If you have trouble identifying target behaviors, refer back to chapter 2 and the goals you set for creating a healthier lifestyle. The intermediate goals you listed there can probably serve as target behaviors.

Rewards Chart

Main goals	Specific target behaviors	Rewards

If you find that your rewards aren't motivating you to change, you may not believe you deserve to be rewarded. In that case, apply the cognitive restructuring techniques in chapters 4 and 6, using them to examine your assumption that you don't deserve to be rewarded. If that doesn't work and your rewards still aren't motivating you to accomplish your target behaviors, you may want to reread the material on the stages of change in chapter 1. You may be stuck in the contemplation stage, in which case you aren't ready to make behavioral changes.

Summary

◆ You deserve to be rewarded.

◆ It's important to choose appropriate rewards.

◆ Even if an activity is enjoyable, it isn't a suitable reward if it encourages unhealthy behaviors.

◆ Rewards can help you succeed in adopting target behaviors that support a healthier lifestyle.

◆ A rewards chart will help you identify target behaviors and choose appropriate rewards for those behaviors.

Chapter 8

Improving Your Sleep

People with bipolar disorder tend to have difficulty sleeping. They may oversleep, not sleep enough, or have poor-quality sleep. One large study of over two thousand people with bipolar disorder found that only 38 percent of them slept normally, without sleep disturbances (Gruber et al. 2009). This is particularly concerning because sleep disturbances may trigger bipolar episodes, contribute to making an episode worse, or both (Harvey 2008). Because of this relationship between sleep and symptoms, regular sleep is particularly important for people with bipolar disorder. In this chapter, I'll review some of the data on why people with bipolar disorder have difficulty sleeping, and I'll offer many strategies that can help you sleep better.

Sleep and Bipolar Disorder

There are probably several reasons why bipolar disorder is associated with poor sleep. One likely reason is that people with bipolar disorder have certain genes that cause abnormalities in the *circadian rhythm system* (Jones, Hare, and Evershed 2005). This system regulates the body's daily biological rhythms, including the rise and fall of body temperature throughout the day and the production of hormones such as melatonin and cortisol. The sleep cycle is affected by these rhythms. For example, body temperature drops as we sleep and levels of melatonin increase. Increased cortisol, on the other hand, is associated with feeling more alert.

Your daily routine of when you go to bed and when you wake up, also known as your sleep-wake cycle, is part of this circadian rhythm system. Thus, the same abnormal genes that cause irregularities in the daily biological rhythms of people with bipolar disorder could also be the cause of their sleep problems. For individuals with bipolar disorder, even changes such as eating a meal late or changing work hours may affect the body's ability to create a normal sleep-wake cycle, due to their genetic vulnerability to circadian rhythm abnormalities (Harvey et al. 2005). This makes it doubly difficult for people with bipolar disorder to keep a stable routine, particularly during times of stress.

People with bipolar disorder are also more likely to have certain nongenetic factors that can contribute to sleep disturbance. For example, stressful life situations have been shown to negatively affect sleep and other symptoms in people with bipolar disorder (Malkoff-Schwartz et al. 1998). Moreover, stress-induced sleep disruptions increase the likelihood that you'll feel more stress, initiating a cycle of increasing stress and disturbed sleep.

Poor sleep is often caused by having negative thoughts about sleep, even among people who don't have bipolar disorder. Sleep-related attitudes and beliefs such as *I won't be able to fall asleep tonight* or *It's after midnight; I'll never fall asleep now* probably contribute to sleep disturbances in people with bipolar disorder (Harvey et al. 2005). People with bipolar disorder also tend to have increased anxiety and fear about their sleeping patterns, false beliefs about sleep, and flawed assumptions about the consequences of disturbed sleep (Plante and Winkelman 2008). This can be a big problem, as having anxious thoughts before bedtime is associated with poor sleep quality (Johnson and Roberts 1995).

In sum, there are both genetic and nongenetic factors that can contribute to sleep difficulties in people with bipolar disorder. The good news is, the nongenetic factors, such as stress, anxiety before bed, and having negative thoughts and false beliefs about sleep, can be corrected. You have the ability to improve your sleep by changing your thoughts. Certain environmental factors and behaviors, from noise to doing overstimulating activities before bed, can also interfere with sleep, and many of these lie within your control as well.

This chapter is dedicated to helping you identify what may be causing any sleep difficulties you're having and coming up with strategies to address those problems. As you'll see, some of the skills you've already learned, such as cognitive restructuring, will be very useful in helping you sleep better.

Sleep Hygiene

You may have heard the term "sleep hygiene." *Sleep hygiene* refers to practices that help people sleep well, as outlined in the following sections.

Keep a Regular Sleep Schedule

Because of the body's circadian rhythm system, people sleep best when they adhere to a regular sleep schedule, such as going to bed at 11 p.m. and waking up at 7 a.m. However, people with bipolar disorder often experience *phase-shifted sleep*, going to bed later and waking up later. For example, you may generally go to bed at 1 a.m. and wake up at 9 a.m. This isn't a problem as long as it doesn't interfere with other things you need to do. The key is to set a regular sleep schedule and stick to it.

Create a Comfortable Sleep Environment

A key aspect of sleep hygiene is having a comfortable sleep environment. Your sleep environment includes anything detectable by one of your five senses: touch, smell, taste, sound, and vision. For touch, make sure that you're wearing comfortable clothes to sleep in that aren't too hot or too cold. It's also important that your bed and bedding be comfortable; for example, switching to flannel sheets in the winter could help with your sleep. Most people find that 65 to 70 degrees is a comfortable temperature for their bedroom. If you're a person who likes to leave a window open to get fresh, cool air, make sure you're still warm enough and comfortable in bed.

As for the other senses, try to ensure that your sleeping space smells good. Although it isn't advisable to burn scented candles or incense while you sleep, you could consider a plug-in air freshener or use a scented fabric softener to wash your pajamas and bedding so that you sleep surrounded by smells that are soothing for you. Then again, you may prefer to have little or no scent in your bedroom; it's very personal. To have a refreshing taste in your mouth, brush your teeth before bed; you might also consider having a mint or not eating just before bed. As for sound, consider whether you like silence while sleeping or sleep better with soothing noise, such as white noise or the sound of rain or the ocean, which can be provided by a white noise or sound machine. Certain sounds can be very soothing, which is why many parents use sound machines to help their babies sleep.

Finally, most people prefer a dark sleeping space, but if you prefer some light, consider getting a night light or cracking the door and keeping a hallway light on. Another consideration is your wake-up time. If your sleep schedule dictates that you wake up early, you may want to leave the curtains open or keep a window cracked to let morning light and noise into your bedroom.

Because you have bipolar disorder, a few modifications to the basic recommendations on sleep environment may be helpful. If you have phase-shifted sleep and that works well in the context of your life, adapt your environment to make sure you can sleep late enough in the morning to get sufficient sleep. Close your curtains or shades before bed so the morning sun doesn't awaken you. If you live on a busy street that gets noisy in the early morning, consider using a white noise machine.

Avoid Stimulants Before Bed

It's important not to get overstimulated before bed. Of course, stimulants, such as caffeine, can make it difficult to sleep. Moreover, using stimulants in the evening may increase the likelihood that you won't stick to your sleep schedule. An obvious recommendation is not consuming caffeine within six hours before bed. Keep in mind that caffeine is present in coffee, chocolate, many teas and energy drinks, and some sodas and pain relievers. Nicotine can be stimulating too, and could also disrupt sleep.

Avoid Alcohol Use

Like many people, you may think that alcohol can help you get to sleep. While it can indeed make you feel tired or drowsy, it actually decreases your overall sleep quality. One way it does this is by reducing the amount of time you spend in REM (rapid eye movement) sleep, a phase of sleep that supports daytime performance and provides energy to the brain and body. Alcohol can also lead to frequent awakenings and generally lighter sleep, rather than the deep, restorative sleep that's so important for your mind and body (Park, Yu, and Ryu 2006). For all of these reasons, sleep disruptions due to drinking alcohol can cause you to feel more tired and sleepy during the day.

Be Thoughtful About When You Exercise

Exercise can be very helpful in promoting good sleep. However, exercise can be stimulating for some people, in part because it causes the body to produce cortisol, which is associated with alertness. The general recommendation is to avoid exercising within three hours of your bedtime. Exercising in the late afternoon may be the best time for promoting sleep without being stimulating too late in the day. However, if you can only exercise earlier in the day, that's fine too.

People with bipolar disorder may need to be especially careful about when they exercise. My colleagues and I recently found that exercise may be associated with mania and hypomania (Sylvia, Friedman, et al. 2013). A likely explanation for this is that people who are manic or hypomanic simply tend to exercise more, as opposed to exercise causing an overly elevated mood. Still, it's best to minimize the chance of sleep problems, so try not to exercise within three hours of your bedtime.

Create a Soothing Bedtime Routine

Beyond avoiding stimulants, alcohol, and exercise before bed, it's also important to avoid other activities that could be stimulating, including watching TV, working, e-mailing, surfing the Internet, and other activities that involve electronic devices. However, everyone is different. These activities could be soothing for you or help you fall asleep. Notice what you do before bed and whether it seems to promote or interfere with sleep. Then make a point of avoiding activities that seem to lead to poor sleep.

Ideally you'll create a soothing bedtime routine. This can signal your body and brain that it's time to go to sleep. For example, every night before bed you might watch a low-key TV show, then shower, take your medications, brush your teeth, and get in bed. In fact, this is especially important for people with bipolar disorder, because sticking to routines can ease bipolar symptoms. And for many people with bipolar disorder, taking medications should be part of an evening routine.

Use Your Bed Only for Sleeping

A key principle of good sleep hygiene is to use your bed only for sleeping. It shouldn't be a place to eat, work, or watch TV. The reason for this is that your bed should signal to you that it's time to sleep, not do activities. The only exception to this is if there's some activity that's very soothing for you to do while lying in bed—something that prepares you for sleep, such as reading. Ideally you'd do this in a comfortable chair, perhaps next to your bed, and then get into bed when you're ready to sleep.

An important aspect of this principle of sleep hygiene is that if you wake up at night and stay awake for more than thirty minutes, you need to get out of bed. You don't want to teach yourself that your bed is a place to be awake—and especially a place to worry about not sleeping! So get out of bed and do something soothing or relaxing for twenty to thirty minutes, then go back to bed. If you don't fall back asleep within thirty minutes, once again get out of bed and do something soothing or relaxing for twenty to thirty minutes. Continue to do this until you fall asleep. This may sound tiring, but that's actually the point.

Because you have bipolar disorder, you're more likely to have negative thoughts about being awake during the night, including during your time out of bed. Practicing cognitive restructuring during the times when you're awake at night will be very helpful.

Eat Lighter Evening Meals and Watch Your Fluid Intake

Eating too soon before bed can cause indigestion. It's generally best to not eat within two or three hours of your bedtime. I've noticed that many people believe they'll have a hard time sleeping if they don't go to bed with a full stomach, but this isn't the case. If you hold this belief, try some cognitive restructuring to convince yourself that you don't need food to fall asleep.

It's so important to drink enough water, and you don't want to wake up thirsty. On the other hand, you don't want to wake up because you need to go to the bathroom, so drink plenty of fluids during the day and taper down in the evening. Be aware that some medications for bipolar disorder, such as lithium, cause dry mouth, which makes people feel thirsty. Keep this side effect in mind so you don't drink too much before bedtime.

Avoid or Limit Naps

Be careful about taking naps. Late-day naps decrease the desire to sleep at night. If you must nap, keep it short, and don't nap later than 5 p.m. That said, the symptoms of depression include fatigue and lack of energy, so people with bipolar disorder may be especially likely to want to nap. If you're very tired and must nap, try to do so at the same time every day and don't nap longer than two hours.

Managing Factors That Make You Vulnerable to Sleep Problems

In the first part of this chapter, we looked at a lot of things that can disrupt sleep. Sometimes these are isolated events, like having an upsetting interaction. Other times they involve choices that you can control, like drinking caffeinated beverages late in the day. And sometimes they're *vulnerabilities*, underlying factors that may be more difficult to change or control. Examples include having bipolar disorder, working at a stressful job, or not having a structured daily routine.

Of course, some of your vulnerabilities may be beyond your direct control, such as genetic predisposition, or family history of depression, or having a loud neighbor. Still, you can often find ways to manage these vulnerabilities. So, let's take a look at some common vulnerabilities to sleep problems among people with bipolar disorder, along with some examples of how to manage them.

Common Vulnerabilities to Sleep Problems and Examples of Ways to Cope

1. Having bipolar disorder

    - Take medications for bipolar disorder.

    - See a therapist.

    - Have a regular routine

    - Get good support from others.

2. Being anxious

    - Consider taking antianxiety medications, seeing a therapist, or both.

    - Use cognitive restructuring; often anxious thoughts aren't accurate.

    - Learn about other anxiety management techniques. There are many, including exercise, yoga, meditation, and deep breathing.

3. Experiencing chronic stress

    - Try to find ways to eliminate or reduce the stress. How can you change the situation?

    - If you can't change the situation, figure out how you can adjust to it more effectively; for example, after interacting with an angry coworker, you might take a break and go for a short walk to blow off steam or do some deep breathing to relax.

4. Having a partner, children, or pets that disrupt your sleep or bedtime routine

- Change the situation if you can. For example, don't allow pets to sleep in your bedroom.

- If your children are disrupting your sleep, help them practice good sleep hygiene too. Everyone will benefit in the short term, and you may help your children avoid future sleep problems.

- If you can't change the situation (for example, your partner snores loudly, but you must share a bedroom), identify what you can do to better manage it, such as wearing earplugs or using a white noise machine.

5. Working the night shift

- Keep a consistent routine, even if it's unusual. This is very important in managing your bipolar disorder.

- Practice good sleep hygiene.

- Consider practicing cognitive restructuring to identify potential false assumptions about your ability to change your schedule.

Chain Analysis

The first step to improving your sleep is knowing what causes your particular sleep problems. Then you'll know which sleep hygiene principles are most important for you to follow. Although there are some general reasons why people with bipolar disorder tend to have poor sleep, everybody has their own unique reasons for not sleeping well. To identify what causes a poor night of sleep for you, you need to give careful thought to what leads up to not sleeping well. A helpful tool for doing this is a *chain analysis*.

A chain analysis can be useful for changing many behaviors, including overeating or not exercising. However, because the topic of this chapter is sleep, all of the examples will relate to sleep problems. A chain analysis is always based on a particular instance of a problem behavior, in this case a certain night of poor sleep. The process involves identifying the sequence of events surrounding the problem behavior. Each event or factor in the sequence is a link in the chain. The first step is identifying any vulnerability that predisposed you to the problem. Next, you determine whether there was a *prompting event*—a trigger that set the stage for the chain to form. Then you identify other links leading up to the problem, listing things that may have been involved in your sleep difficulty. Next, you examine the *consequences*, looking at the impacts of having a poor night of sleep. Finally, you choose a new behavior, being sure to set specific, realistic goals as you do so. The following figure depicts a chain analysis, with "Behavior" being a poor night of sleep.

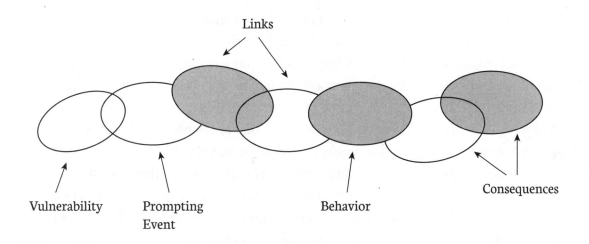

Shortly, I'll guide you through a chain analysis for your own sleep difficulties. But first, to illustrate the process, let's consider an example.

Emily was diagnosed with bipolar disorder several years ago, and as far back as she can remember, she's had trouble with her sleep. As a result, she believes that she'll never be able to sleep well and that she'll never get to sleep before the early morning hours. Based on these beliefs, she tends to stay up very late, often until 2 or 3 a.m., watching TV and surfing the Internet. Emily tends to eat late at night too because she thinks she can't fall asleep without having a full stomach. Early every morning she's woken up by her dog, who needs to be fed and let outside. So on average, Emily only gets five or six hours of sleep. Therefore, she thinks she can't get through her day without drinking lots of coffee to keep her awake. On many days, Emily drinks a 16-ounce coffee as late as 6 p.m.

Because of her sleep schedule, Emily often doesn't have time for some very basic self-care activities, like showering, brushing her teeth, and eating breakfast. Her first meal is typically lunch—another reason Emily believes she needs a snack late at night. So her meal schedule is skewed too, with mealtimes typically being noon, 7 p.m., and midnight. When she's had a particularly bad night of sleep, Emily finds that she's more irritable the next day, has difficulty focusing at work, and feels even more convinced that she'll never be able to sleep well.

Step 1. Identifying Vulnerabilities

To determine what could be causing Emily's sleep problems and how she might solve them, let's do a chain analysis. Of course, before doing a chain analysis you have to identify the problem behavior. In Emily's case, and throughout this chapter, the problem is sleeping poorly. Once you've selected the problem to solve, you can begin the actual process of a chain analysis, looking at everything involved in it. The first step is to identify vulnerabilities: the underlying factors that make the problem more likely.

Vulnerabilities are usually bigger-picture things that are harder to change, so they typically aren't specific to a given day, week, or event. Rather, they're factors that have been present for a while, such as your job, your long-term beliefs, your partner, your medications, your pets, your medical diagnoses, or your medical or family history. However, sometimes they can be changed or managed more effectively (as previously discussed), so it's useful to know what they are. Returning to Emily's example, here are a few factors that could be considered vulnerabilities.

Vulnerabilities:

- *Having bipolar disorder*

- *Believing she can't sleep*

- *Having a dog*

Step 2. Identifying a Prompting Event

The second step in doing a chain analysis is to see if there was a prompting event: a specific situation that may have triggered the problem. For example, perhaps a friend was visiting and kept Emily up, maybe Emily had a conflict with a coworker, maybe she has the flu, or perhaps a neighbor's new dog barked all night. These are just a few examples of the kinds of things that can be prompting events. However, in Emily's example it doesn't seem that there were any unusual, specific events that caused her sleep difficulty.

Prompting event:

- *None*

Step 3. Identifying Other Links Leading Up to the Problem

The next step is to identify any other events or elements of daily life that could have contributed to the problem. For this part of the chain analysis, it's important to be very thoughtful about any factors that could be involved. Typically, you should be able to identify at least five links in a chain leading up to the problem. In Emily's case, she may not see that certain parts of her routine are contributing to her sleep disturbance. These links may be more obvious to other people, so she might consider seeking input from someone she trusts.

Links leading up to the problem:

- *Having negative thoughts about sleep:*

  - *"I need food in order to sleep."*

  - *"I won't fall asleep before 2 or 3 a.m."*

  - *"I must have eight hours of sleep to be rested."*

- *Staying up late*

- *Doing stimulating activities, like surfing the web, late at night*

- *Eating late*

- *Having a dog that barks in the morning*

- *Not eating in the morning*

- *Not having a good morning routine*

- *Drinking a lot of coffee, especially late in the day*

Step 4. Examining the Consequences of the Problem Behavior

The next step is to identify the consequences of the problem behavior. This can provide a lot of motivation for changing the behavior. In Emily's case, there are many negative consequences to not sleeping well. Here are just a few examples of the effects her difficulty sleeping may have on her life.

Consequences:

- *Increased irritability*

- *Impaired concentration*

- *Increased vulnerability to sleeping poorly due to strengthened beliefs that she won't be able to sleep*

Step 5. Choosing a New Behavior

Obviously Emily wants to sleep better, but if she's to make progress in that direction, she needs to set specific, realistic goals. There are many possibilities for Emily. Here are just a few.

New behavior:

- *Setting a sleep schedule of getting to bed by midnight and getting up at 8 a.m.*

- *Establishing a morning routine that involves basic self-care and breakfast*

- *Eating dinner by 10 p.m.*

Using a Chain Analysis to Make Changes

Hopefully Emily's example showed you how a chain analysis can help you really understand the factors involved in a problem. This is the goal of a chain analysis: doing a very detailed assessment of a problem so you can understand what's contributing to the difficulty. A good chain analysis will also help you choose appropriate new behaviors and provide motivation for adopting these new behaviors. In this way, it will allow you to be much more effective in making the necessary changes to your thoughts and behaviors. Let's consider another example of someone who has difficulty sleeping. This time, we'll really focus on how a chain analysis can be useful in making changes.

Linda, who has bipolar disorder, had been struggling to manage her irritability and erratic behavior at work. Ultimately, she was fired because her boss had doubts about the soundness of her decision making and her ability to be a team player. After losing her job, Linda started having a lot of trouble sleeping. Now she lies awake at night in bed worrying about how she can find another job so she'll be able to pay her bills.

Because Linda no longer has a reason to get up in the morning, she's started staying in bed until 1 p.m. Feeling tired and depressed and not having a full schedule, Linda often watches TV for hours on end during the day and doesn't get around to things that she needs to do, such as working on her résumé, looking for a new job, or paying her bills. Before she was fired, Linda had been walking with a coworker during her lunch hour. Now, without her job to provide that structure, she's quit exercising. In addition, she's started overeating to distract herself from her feelings of anxiety and sadness.

Despite not having energy during the day, Linda doesn't go to bed until very late because she has trouble turning off her brain at night. She dreads bedtime, when her mind races with anxious thoughts about finding a new job. To make matters worse, now Linda has started worrying that she won't be able to get to sleep. She fears her sleep problems will deepen her mood problems and make it even more difficult for her to find a new job.

You may be thinking that there are probably many reasons why Linda isn't feeling very good other than just her difficulty sleeping. I agree. But Linda's sleep problems are impacting other areas of her life, especially because she has bipolar disorder. If she can improve her sleep, it's likely that she'll start feeling better and be more effective in other areas of her life. So let's do a chain analysis for Linda's sleep difficulties, taking a close look at what she might do differently. As you'll see, there are many ways to manage the events and other factors that form the links in the chain.

Step 1. Identifying and Managing Vulnerabilities

Once you've identified vulnerabilities, you can begin to manage them. In Linda's case, having bipolar disorder is her primary vulnerability. Here are a few ideas on how she might manage this.

Vulnerability: *Having bipolar disorder, especially depression*

Ways to manage this vulnerability:

- *Take her medications.*

- *See her therapist.*

- *Get extra support or help from friends and family members.*

Step 2. Identifying and Managing Prompting Events

Linda's prompting event was losing her job—something that's already happened and therefore can't be managed. Still, she can consider what she might have done differently to prevent it from happening. Other types of prompting events can be managed, such as having a conflict with your boss. For these, it's highly worthwhile to come up with strategies to work with them.

Prompting event: *Getting fired*

Ways to manage the prompting event:

- *Take time off from work when she feels stressed.*

- *Get extra support at work.*

- *Look for a job that's a better fit.*

- *Get more support for managing her bipolar disorder, such as therapy, a medication change, or talking to a friend.*

Step 3. Identifying and Managing Other Links Leading Up to the Problem

The next step is to identify other links leading up to the problem and come up with ways to manage them. As you'll see from the example completed for Linda below, the principles of sleep hygiene discussed at the beginning of this chapter can be particularly useful.

Link	Ways to manage the link
Lying in bed awake for hours	*Get out of bed after thirty minutes if she hasn't been able to sleep.*
Not exercising	*Gradually get more active again by doing things she usually enjoys, such as walking at the mall.*
Not having a good daily routine	*Create a daily routine, perhaps by volunteering, seeing friends, walking her parents' dog, and setting aside specific times to work on her job search.*
Eating too close to bedtime	*Eat dinner before 8 p.m.*
Not having a good bedtime routine	*Create a bedtime routine. For example, she might spend twenty minutes writing and responding to e-mail, then shower, take her medications, read a magazine, brush her teeth, and, finally, go to bed.*
Having negative thoughts: *"I'll never find another job."* *"I won't be able to fall asleep."* *"I need to eat to fall asleep."*	*Practice cognitive restructuring to identify the evidence against negative thoughts and come up new, alternative thoughts.*

Step 4. Examining and Managing the Consequences of the Problem Behavior

As mentioned, being aware of the consequences of a problem behavior can provide a lot of motivation to change the behavior. As you begin practicing your new behaviors, the consequences should diminish, but sometimes this may take a while. In the meanwhile, you can often manage troublesome consequences. Some of the key consequences of Linda's sleep problems are lack of energy, difficulty focusing, and trouble looking for a new job. Here are some ideas of how she might manage each.

Consequence	Ways to manage the consequence
Lack of energy	*Plan engaging activities that will keep her busy.*
Difficulty focusing	*Take a short break from time to time.* *Reward herself for accomplishing tasks that require focus.*
Trouble looking for a new job	*Ask a friend to review her résumé.* *Use the goal-setting approach in chapter 2 to create a plan with specific steps.*

Step 5. Choosing New Behaviors

Again, it's important to set specific, realistic goals. So even though Linda's overall goal is simply to sleep better, she needs to be specific when choosing new behaviors to replace the problem behavior. The ways to manage the links in the chain identified in step 3 can come in handy here.

New behaviors

- *Eat dinner before 8 p.m.*

- *Create a bedtime routine and follow it.*

- *Get to bed by midnight.*

- *Get out of bed after thirty minutes if she hasn't been able to sleep.*

- *Practice cognitive restructuring with her negative thoughts.*

Exercise: Doing a Chain Analysis for Your Sleep Problems

Based on Emily's and Linda's examples, you now have a good idea of how a chain analysis works—and how helpful it can be. Now it's your turn to do a chain analysis. Because this approach is so helpful, I strongly encourage you to go through all of the steps. If sleep isn't an issue for you, that's fine. You can apply this approach to any problem behavior.

The instructions below will guide you through your chain analysis step by step. After the instructions, you'll find a blank worksheet to use throughout the process. (A downloadable version of this worksheet, useful for chain analyses you might do for other problem behaviors in the future, is available at http://www.newharbinger.com/31304; see the back of the book for instructions on how to access it.) One final note before we get started: If you get stuck at any point in the process, especially in steps 3 through 5, consider revisiting chapter 1 to read about the stages of change. You might also consider seeking help from a friend or therapist.

Step 1. Identify and Manage Your Vulnerabilities

The first step in creating your chain analysis is to identify your vulnerabilities. What makes you more likely to have sleep problems? Earlier in the chapter, I mentioned some of the most common vulnerabilities among my clients with bipolar disorder. Those vulnerabilities are listed below. Check any that apply to you, then write those statements in the "Vulnerabilities" section of the worksheet. Also write any other vulnerabilities that apply to you.

_____ Having bipolar disorder

_____ Working the night shift

_____ Having a partner, children, or pets that disrupt your sleep or bedtime routine

_____ Being anxious

_____ Having parents with insomnia, anxiety, or mood disorders

_____ Experiencing chronic stress

_____ Taking certain medications

_____ Living in a noisy environment, such as near a highway, or having a loud neighbor

_____ Needing to travel a lot, especially to different time zones

_____ Other: _____

_____ Other: _____

Once you've identified your vulnerabilities, it's time to come up with strategies for managing them. In the section on vulnerabilities earlier in this chapter, I outlined some approaches that may be helpful for vulnerabilities to sleep problems. So if sleep issues are the problem you're examining here, you may want to revisit that section.

Step 2. Identify and Manage the Prompting Event

The next step in creating your chain analysis is to identify whether a recent life event may have caused your sleep difficulties. If your sleep problems are chronic, there may not be a prompting event. However, even relatively minor events, such as being late to work because of traffic or having a disagreement with a friend, could be a prompting event. So give some serious thought to whether anything happened recently that could have impacted your sleep. If you identify a prompting event, write it below "Prompting event" in the worksheet. Then try to think of ways to decrease the likelihood that it will happen again. Record what you come up with on the worksheet.

Step 3. Identify and Manage Other Links Leading Up to the Problem

The most challenging part of your chain analysis will probably be identifying all of the things that happened that may have contributed to the problem. As you identify these links, write them on the worksheet under "Links leading up to the problem." If you can't identify at least five such links, you'll probably benefit from seeking input from others. Another tip is to experiment. For example, if you aren't sure whether sleeping with your blinds up impacts your sleep, try closing them one night. If you aren't sure whether staring at your alarm clock prevents you from sleeping, try turning it away from your bed and see if that helps you sleep. Once you've identified links leading up to the problem, you can work on managing them. Write all of your ideas about managing each link on the worksheet.

Step 4. Examine and Manage the Consequences of the Problem Behavior

As mentioned, understanding the consequences of a problem behavior can help motivate you to adopt the new behavior you'll choose in step 5, and to make other changes in order to better manage earlier links in the chain. For example, Linda may be much more motivated to make changes to her lifestyle and routine to sleep better once she sees that her sleep problems are impacting her ability to look for a new job.

People often report that they feel very irritable, distracted, and emotional when they don't sleep well. These are consequences that are unpleasant for anyone, but because you may already be experiencing these symptoms as a result of bipolar disorder, these consequences may heighten symptoms that are already difficult and interfering with your life. This is one reason why it's so important to make whatever changes are needed to ensure you get better sleep. To keep the consequences in mind, write them on the worksheet under "Consequences." Then, because it may take you a while to implement your new behaviors or for these new behaviors to have an effect on other parts of your life, take some time to brainstorm ways to manage each consequence.

Step 5. Choose a New Behavior

Finally, in the last section of the worksheet, labeled "Problem behavior," write the behavior that's causing difficulty. Then choose one or more new behaviors to replace the old, problematic behavior and write them under "New behaviors." These new behaviors are goals, so make sure they're specific and realistic. (If you aren't sure how to make them specific and realistic, revisit chapter 2.) So, "sleeping better" isn't a good new goal because it isn't specific enough. How do you want to sleep better? Do you want to get to bed earlier? Do you want to stop sleeping so late that your day gets off to a stressful start? As a reminder, many of the ideas you've come up with for managing the links that precede the problem behavior may be appropriate new target behaviors.

Chain Analysis Worksheet

Vulnerabilities	Ways to manage these vulnerabilities
Prompting event	Ways to manage the prompting event
Links leading up to the problem	Ways to manage these links

Consequences	Ways to manage these consequences

Problem behavior	New behaviors

Doing a chain analysis is somewhat involved, but for problem behaviors that are having a significant negative impact on your life, it's well worth the effort. And as you come up with ways to manage various links, you may find that you overcome many difficulties beyond just the problem behavior you originally targeted. Throughout, remember that realistic and specific goals are crucial. In addition to making your goals achievable, this will ensure that you can determine whether you're actually succeeding in making the changes you've chosen.

If you follow through on the behavior changes and management strategies outlined in the chain analysis and the problem doesn't improve, you probably haven't identified all of the links contributing to the problem. Go back and look for any missing links so that you can break the chain. Also consider seeking help from a therapist or a trusted friend.

Summary

- Sleep problems are common among people with bipolar disorder.

- Improving your sleep can help you manage your bipolar disorder.

- You can control and improve your sleep.

- Doing a chain analysis can help you understand the reasons for your sleep problems and will also help you come up with solutions:

  - Once you know your vulnerabilities, you can manage them.

  - Identifying the links leading up to your sleep problems will help you understand and solve your sleep problems.

  - Knowing the consequences of your sleep difficulties can provide motivation to make the changes necessary for sleeping better.

  - Setting specific, realistic goals for new behaviors is essential for success.

Chapter 9

Making Good Decisions

Making good decisions is the cornerstone to creating a healthier lifestyle. Every day you're faced with numerous decisions about what to do, many with a bearing on your wellness: what to eat and drink, when to eat and drink, and how much to consume; whether to be active, what to do, and how intensely or for how long; when to wake up and go to sleep, and how to structure your daily routine. The list goes on and on. Each of these decisions has a bearing on whether you're creating a more healthy lifestyle. So in this chapter, I'll focus on two key skills that can help you make better decisions: bringing more awareness to your decision-making process, and understanding and managing your cravings.

Bringing More Awareness to Decision Making

In this chapter, when I say "awareness," I mean consciously and mindfully observing things, particularly your behavior, the choices before you, and the reasons why a certain choice may be better or worse for you. We tend to think we're aware of what we're doing, or of most things we do, but often we aren't actually observing our experience or describing it to ourselves.

Driving is a great example. How observant are you when you're driving? Do you feel the steering wheel in your hands or the pressure of your feet on the pedals? Do you take note of all the signs and landmarks you pass along the way? Or do you sometimes find yourself at your destination with little or no recollection of the drive? People often find that they've driven with very little awareness and were instead caught up in thoughts: compiling a grocery list, rehearsing for a meeting that they're driving to, rehashing a difficult interaction, and on and on.

Here's another example—one more closely aligned with wellness. Luke and Paul are both having a late night snack of crackers and peanut butter. As Luke eats his snack, he has thoughts along these lines: *These crackers are really good. I like the way the peanut butter adds flavor to the cracker and how the texture of the smooth, creamy peanut butter contrasts with the crunchy cracker. I wish I had plans tonight, but I'm really enjoying this snack.*

And here's a sample of Paul's thoughts: *I feel so lonely. I can't believe I have nothing to do tonight. I'm such a loser. Wow, I've almost finished this box of crackers… I wonder why I never have any plans. I have to make plans for tomorrow night.*

Who do you think is bringing more awareness to eating his snack, Luke or Paul? Clearly, Luke is more aware of what he's eating and more in the present moment than Paul. It seems as though Paul barely notices that he's eating because he's focusing on so many other things. Paul doesn't seem to be observing his experience of eating or describing his experience to himself, which reduces his overall awareness of eating.

Noticing Decision Points

Awareness is a crucial foundation for making good choices. You need to observe your experience closely enough to know when you face a decision or are about to make a choice. Once you know that, you have the opportunity to deliberately choose what you want to do. For example, if both Luke and Paul were trying to eat fewer calories, who would be in a better position to eat fewer crackers and peanut butter? To answer this question, consider which of them might be more aware that he's putting cracker after cracker in his mouth. It seems that Luke, who's actively observing his experience of eating, would be more likely to stop eating before Paul, because Paul is eating rather mindlessly.

Making Decisions Consciously

Let's look at a few examples of people who have set certain goals for adopting a healthier lifestyle. As you read each story, consider whether the person is showing much awareness of what he or she is doing. Also consider whether each is likely to make good decisions that support his or her goals.

Maria

Goal: Maria, who's single, has a goal of eating smaller portion sizes.

Scenario: Maria doesn't like to cook, so she often has dinner at a local restaurant on her way home from work. Because she's alone, she usually brings a book to read while eating dinner. When a friend asked what she had for dinner last night, Maria struggled to remember what she'd eaten because she'd been so into her book.

Awareness: Was Maria aware of her behavior while eating? No, she clearly wasn't. She had trouble remembering what she ate.

Likelihood of good decision making: So, is Maria likely to make good decisions to support her goal of eating smaller portions? Given that she isn't aware of what she's eating, it's unlikely that she's paying careful attention to how much she's eating.

Ted

Goal: Ted is trying to improve his health by getting more active, so he's set a goal of walking faster and for longer distances.

Scenario: Recently when he was out walking, Ted used his iPod to listen to music. He found himself singing along to the tunes and swinging his arms and legs in rhythm with the music, which really pushed his pace. His mind sometimes wandered to other things, but he tried to keep his focus on walking—which wasn't too hard, because pushing the pace was putting some strain on his legs and making him breathe faster.

Awareness: Was Ted aware of his behavior while walking? Yes. He may have sometimes tuned in to other things while walking, but overall he was closely observing how it felt to be walking.

Likelihood of good decision making: Is Ted likely to make good decisions to support his goal of walking faster and for longer distances? Definitely. Ted has a good sense of how far and fast he's walking, and he can base his decision on that awareness.

Monica

Goal: Monica wants to drink less, and she's set a goal of not stopping at a bar on her way home from work.

Scenario: One day at work, she has a fight with her coworker Lucy. She couldn't believe that Lucy submitted an inaccurate time sheet that didn't account for an entire day off. Worse, Lucy tried to deny it when Monica confronted her about it. As Monica drives home from work fuming about the incident, she's almost entirely unaware of the drive and ultimately finds herself pulling up at a bar in her neighborhood. Since she's already there, she figures she might as well stop in for a drink to blow off steam.

Awareness: Was Monica aware of her behavior while driving? No. Monica isn't thinking about where she's going, and once she gets to the bar, she remains focused on the fight with her coworker.

Likelihood of good decision making: Is Monica likely to make good decisions to support her goal of not stopping in at the bar on her way home? Again, no. Monica is so focused on the conflict with Lucy that she chooses to go in for a drink, rather than turning her mind to her goal and why it's important to her.

Owen

Goal: Owen has sleep problems and has set a goal of going to bed by midnight.

Scenario: Owen thinks watching movies will help him relax, but once he starts watching in the evening, he gets so caught up in the excitement that he often watches several movies in a row. He eventually falls asleep on the couch and often has no idea what time he fell asleep.

Awareness: Is Owen aware of his behavior around his bedtime routine? No, he isn't. He's so focused on what he's watching that he loses track of the need for a good bedtime routine.

Likelihood of good decision making: Is Owen likely to make good decisions to support his goal of going to bed by midnight? Again, no. Currently, Owen usually has no idea when he falls asleep.

Cindy

Goal: Cindy wants to lose weight and has set a goal of losing one pound every two weeks. And because she really enjoys food, she's also decided to relish every single bite of her meals in the hopes that this will make her feel more satisfied.

Scenario: Cindy especially enjoys international cuisine. One night she went to an Indian restaurant. She noticed that the rice was a bit undercooked and chewy, but the vegetable curry was wonderful, with such complex and interesting spices. She could detect a few specific spices, like turmeric and cumin, but there were other flavors she couldn't identify. After savoring every bite of her dinner, she decided to treat herself to dessert and ordered rice pudding. It was wonderfully rich and creamy, but after a few bites, she realized she was really full. Regretfully, she pushed the rest of her dessert aside and asked for her check.

Awareness: Is Cindy aware of her behavior around eating? Emphatically yes! Cindy is extremely aware of what she's eating.

Likelihood of good decision making: Is Cindy likely to make good decisions to support her goal of losing one pound every two weeks? Again, emphatically yes. Cindy's focus on the foods she eats and how they make her feel will help her make good decisions about what to eat.

How Bipolar Disorder Affects Decision Making

Bringing greater awareness to what you're doing and describing it to yourself can greatly increase the likelihood that you'll make choices to support a healthier lifestyle. If you allow yourself to see the decisions you're making, you'll be in a much better position to make them consciously. However, there are two symptoms of bipolar disorder that can make it difficult for you to be aware of what you're doing and opt for healthy choices: lack of insight, and impulsivity.

By *insight*, I mean being aware of the effects or consequences of your actions. For example, if you have a goal to lose weight, you'd be showing good insight if you understood that you tend to have difficulty eating healthy foods at Mexican restaurants and decided to eat at these restaurants less often. Someone with poor insight, on the other hand, might just keep eating at Mexican restaurants whenever the urge strikes.

Unfortunately, being depressed or having an elevated or manic mood can stand in the way of good insight. In these mood states, people's thinking often becomes overly negative or positive—so much so that they lose the ability to think too far in advance. And when you can't think in advance, you can't connect your current actions with later consequences of these actions. For this reason, having bipolar disorder means you have to try to be very aware of what you're doing in each moment (for example, drinking coffee or a caffeinated soda in the evening) and how it could affect what you want to do later (sleep better at night).

Impulsivity is related. It means acting without giving much thought to what you're doing. As you might imagine, being impulsive can make it difficult to have good insight. For example, say you see a doughnut when you're feeling impulsive. You're probably likely to eat it right away. But what if you were to stop and think about that doughnut for thirty seconds, or even just five? Do you think that by the time you counted to five, you might be able to resist eating that doughnut? This is the difference between being impulsive and being insightful. In a way, this is great news. Think about it: stopping for just five seconds before making a decision might greatly reduce your impulsivity and help you make better decisions.

That said, because you have bipolar disorder, you're simply more likely to be impulsive, particularly when you're depressed or manic. It's important to be especially patient with yourself when you do something you didn't really want to do, like dive right in and eat the doughnut, because making good decisions can be harder for you. However, by applying yourself to becoming more deliberate, such as by counting to five before making a decision, you can learn to make better, more health-promoting choices.

How to Practice Awareness

Here are a few tips that will help you practice more awareness, which, ultimately, will improve your insight and decrease your impulsivity.

Start simple. Think of a situation you already bring a fair amount of awareness to, whether petting your cat or drinking a cup of coffee first thing in the morning. Then, next time you do that activity, focus on all of your senses: How does your cat's fur feel? Can you hear your cat purring? Do you see steam rising from the coffee? As you bring the cup of coffee to your mouth, can you smell its aroma? How does it taste?

Observe and describe. Find a time when you aren't rushed and simply describe what you see around you and what you're doing. You might be in your office, walking in a park, lying in your bed—the possibilities are endless. Simply making a point of observing what's around you and what you're doing, then describing your experience to yourself, can greatly increase your capacity for awareness.

Begin with positive experiences. It's generally more enjoyable to practice awareness during positive experiences. So look for opportunities to practice awareness when doing things you enjoy. Say you like going to the beach. Next time you go, mentally describe your experience, calling on all of your senses. Describe the sound of the waves, how the sun or breeze feels, and what you see. Can you smell the salt in the air, or maybe even taste it a bit?

Remember that you cannot fail. As you know, having bipolar disorder means you're more prone to negative thoughts, so you may have negative thoughts about your ability to practice awareness. To challenge these potential negative thoughts, keep this in mind: You cannot fail at this task because you're just trying to *increase* your awareness. It would be unrealistic to assume that you can practice awareness at all times, so instead work to acknowledge the times when you are more aware. You might even reward yourself for this from time to time.

All of these techniques for practicing awareness will increase your ability to notice decision points and think before doing something. This can go a long way toward reducing impulsivity. Although bipolar disorder can make it more challenging to use insight and make thoughtful decisions, you can do it!

Monitoring Your Mood

Given that bringing awareness to your decisions depends on your mood, a useful tool in making good decisions is tracking your mood. This is particularly important for people with bipolar disorder because of their mood-related symptoms. You can track your mood by using a scale of 0 to 5 to rate the intensity of your mood. On this scale, 0 means a mood state isn't present, 1 means it's mild, 3 means it's moderate, and 5 means it's severe or extreme.

Mood Tracking Chart

Day	Depression	Elevated mood
Monday	1	2
Tuesday	2	2
Wednesday	3	3
Thursday	4	1
Friday	5	0
Saturday	4	0
Sunday	3	0

I highly recommend that you track your mood every day, using a chart like the one shown here. This will not only help you make better decisions but also teach you about patterns in your moods. For example, you might begin to notice that you can generally make good decisions when your depression is between 0 and 3, but that it's difficult to do so if your mood is elevated at all, even just to 1, or mild, on the scale.

There are also many ways to track your mood electronically through online programs or phone apps. These tools can be especially useful because they often allow you to track other things, including physical activity, medications, sleep, and anxiety, along with notes or comments on each day. If you use one of these programs or apps, you can share your log-in information or send your mood tracking data to anyone on your support team, especially your doctors. These apps and programs store your data for many months or even longer, allowing you to easily track how you're doing over time without relying on a lot of paper, as written mood tracking does. I'm not an expert in phone apps, but here are a few suggestions among the many options available:

- **iMoodJournal.** With this app you can record your mood, thoughts, sleep patterns, and medications. It has a reminder function that prompts you to log in and record how you're doing.

- **eMoods.** This app allows you to input emotional highs and lows of the day, along with other symptoms, and jot notes about your day. It will also help you track your sleep habits and medications.

- **T2 Mood Tracker.** This app includes a full range of mood scales, or you can build your own scales to record how you're doing. It can show your data in the form of graphs.

- **Optimism.** With this app you can record your daily moods and symptoms. Like T2 Mood Tracker, it can display your data visually. It can also be set up to send you reports by e-mail.

To highlight the impact of mood on making decisions, there are two rules I generally encourage my clients with bipolar disorder to use. The first is to not make big decisions when you aren't feeling well. These would be any decisions that could have a moderate to major impact on your life, such as buying a new computer, deciding to skip work, or ignoring a friend. Wait until you feel better to make any big decisions. The truth is, most decisions can be put off for a few days or a week, or even longer if need be.

The second rule is to seek advice from two trusted people about any decisions you make when you aren't feeling well. If both people agree with your decision, it's probably okay to proceed. However, if even just one person doesn't agree with your decision, you need to put the decision aside until later, when you're feeling better.

The next section covers dealing with emotional decisions around cravings. Monitoring your mood can be extremely helpful with these kinds of decisions.

Cravings

A *craving* is a powerful, urgent desire for something—often something that isn't healthy. Just about everyone craves something. Some people may crave cigarettes or alcohol, others may crave buying new things, and yet others may crave foods like candy or pizza. Both depressed mood and elevated mood can lead to cravings that interfere with making healthy choices. Researchers have found that a negative mood can increase the desire for unhealthy foods (Hepworth et al. 2010). In my practice, I've found that many of my clients say they prefer creamy or sweet comfort foods when their mood is depressed, believing that these foods can help put them in a better mood.

Of course, when you're depressed it's usually harder to find the motivation necessary to resist cravings and make decisions that support a healthy lifestyle. Yet mania or an elevated mood can also interfere with making healthy choices and may also increase certain kinds of cravings. For example, you may find that you crave having specific things or doing particular activities, both of which can lead to poor decisions about spending money, calling people at strange hours, or being distracted at work. Cravings to do or say things when you're manic can be very problematic, so it's particularly important to be thoughtful about the decisions that you make when your mood is elevated.

Keep in mind that having a mood episode doesn't mean you'll definitely make unhealthy choices. It just means you're more likely to. Therefore, you need to be proactive about monitoring your mood so you'll have a better understanding of when you're more likely to make unhealthy choices. For this reason, it's a good idea to monitor your mood as discussed in the last section, just as you've been monitoring your diet and activity level. Again, the more aware you are of your current mood, the more likely it is that you can notice cravings and desires to make unhealthy choices and then decide to do something different.

In the sections that follow, I'll cover some of the cravings most common among people with bipolar disorder: cravings for food, sleep, substances, and buying new things. As you can see from that list, it's possible to crave something you sometimes genuinely need (food or sleep) or something you don't need (substances or an excessive number of new things). Awareness is the key to sorting out what you truly need and what you don't, so let's take a look at each of those categories and how to bring awareness to cravings for each.

Food

Of course, a certain amount of food is necessary for survival. So how can you know if a craving for food represents a real need? Thankfully, it's fairly simple to figure out. Women only need about 1,500 to 1,800 calories per day, and men need approximately 1,800 to 2,000 calories per day. Of course, actual daily calorie needs vary from person to person, but the majority of people will do just fine eating this number of calories, and some people may need even fewer. (But do consult a doctor before eating less than this on an ongoing basis.) Keeping a food diary or using a diet tracking app, as discussed in chapter 4, can help you to monitor your daily calorie intake. If you don't do a lot of physical activity but are consuming much more than the number of calories mentioned above, chances are that any food cravings don't stem from a genuine need for food.

Food cravings are very common. Nearly everyone has them, regardless of whether they have bipolar disorder. However, as discussed, your bipolar illness makes it likely that you'll have more cravings and have more difficulty managing them. If food cravings are an issue for you, be sure to read the section on managing cravings closely.

Sleep

As with food, a certain amount of sleep is necessary for survival. So if you feel like you're craving sleep, you may just need more sleep or be sleep deprived. If so, your body is simply telling you that you aren't getting enough sleep. However, you may also crave sleep when you don't need it. This often happens when people are depressed. You may be sleeping ten or fourteen hours a day, or even longer, and still want more sleep. This is because depression is characterized by feelings of fatigue or tiredness. Your body literally wants to rest when it doesn't need to.

To help you figure out whether you need more sleep, monitor how many hours of sleep you're getting. Most people need seven to eight hours of sleep to feel rested, but it can vary depending on the person. You may also need more sleep if you've recently been sleep deprived. If you experience episodes of mania or elevated mood due to bipolar disorder, you've probably experienced periods of insomnia. This sleep deprivation during mania often means you'll have to catch up on sleep after a manic episode or want to sleep more than usual.

For the sake of your health, do what you can to get enough sleep, but not too much, on a regular basis. One review of many sleep studies found that either sleeping less than five hours or more than nine hours on average increases the risk of death (Cappuccio et al. 2010). This suggests that if you're craving more than nine hours of sleep on a regular basis, you're probably experiencing a craving for something you don't need.

Substances

Substances such as alcohol, drugs, or cigarettes are not required by your body to survive. Therefore, it's important to find strategies for overcoming these cravings. If you've ever experienced withdrawing from a substance, you may be tempted to disagree. During withdrawal, it really feels like your body needs the alcohol, cigarette, or other substance to survive. This is what happens when your body gets physiologically dependent on a substance. But even in this case, it's possible to withdraw from the substance, provided you take the appropriate measures to stay safe. Then you'll see that your body no longer needs that substance to function, and that you actually function better without it.

Avoiding alcohol is particularly important for people with bipolar disorder, who are more likely to abuse alcohol than the general population (Grant et al. 2006). Alcohol can also have harmful interactions with some medications used to treat the illness. In addition, it can worsen the course of bipolar disorder. For example, one study found that alcohol use was correlated with increased psychiatric hospitalizations (Cassidy, Ahearn, and Carroll 2001). The situation is similar for smoking, which has been linked to heightened symptoms, increased suicidality, and poorer functioning in people with bipolar disorder (Ostacher et al. 2006).

Buying New Things

Some people crave buying new things. If you experience this, try asking yourself whether something you want to buy is necessary for your survival. I bet 99 percent of the time, you could survive without buying that new thing. Of course, I'm not talking about things like food, medications, basic toiletries, and so on. The things I'm talking about are along the lines of electronics, furniture, knickknacks, gifts, unneeded clothes, and other items that might be considered extras or luxuries, rather than necessities.

The craving to buy new things can be very strong, and it's also quite common, including among people who don't have bipolar disorder. However, the desire to buy new things can be especially compelling for people with bipolar disorder because "retail therapy" can actually work to improve mood in the short run. For a while, you may feel better because of having something new. But how long does that feeling last? And when it wears off, you're likely to want some other new thing, leading to an unsustainable cycle of spending. As a result, people who give in to the craving to buy new things may end up in debt.

Managing Cravings

To manage your cravings, you need to increase your awareness of what you actually need and what you don't need. Then you need to learn to feel more comfortable with the craving. The rest of this chapter will help you do that.

Exercise: Using a Cravings Intensity Scale

One way to increase your awareness of your cravings is to create a cravings intensity scale. This will help you tune in to when you experience cravings and why. This is crucial information for controlling or resisting cravings. The easiest and clearest way to explain this exercise is with an example, so I've provided one. Then, after the example, you'll find a blank worksheet for your use. If you crave several things (certain foods, cigarettes, sleep, caffeine, alcohol, substances, new things), complete a Cravings Intensity Worksheet for each type of craving, using the downloadable version of this worksheet available at http://www.newharbinger.com/31304. (See the back of the book for instructions on how to access it.)

Sample Cravings Intensity Worksheet

Discomfort level	Description and examples
0 No discomfort	I experience almost no cravings when I'm watching TV right after a meal.
1	After a meal, I might have a very slight craving if I smell foods I like.
2	An hour after I've eaten, I may start to have slight cravings, especially if I see or smell my favorite foods.
3 Mild discomfort	When I'm around my friends, I tend not to eat because I'm embarrassed, so I usually eat just before seeing them. But if they're eating I have mild cravings.
4	After I walk my dog, I start thinking I deserve a snack because I just did some exercise. This creates slightly stronger cravings.
5	A couple of hours after a meal, I start to think that maybe it could be time to eat again. I think about what snacks I have on hand or what might be good to eat.
6 Moderate discomfort	Just before I go out, I feel as though I need to eat something because I'm embarrassed about eating in front of others. Before leaving the house, I have a hard time resisting the urge to eat.
7	In the evening, I often feel depressed. At those times I tend to think a lot about food and plan what I could eat, which creates some fairly strong cravings.
8	If I haven't eaten in several hours, I start thinking that I have to eat something or I might get shaky. I think it's time for a meal or that I deserve to eat something and it's very hard to resist.
9	At night I feel very alone and think there's no meaning to my life. I often have terrible cravings for something to fill me up.
10 Severe discomfort	If I have a day of eating poorly and don't exercise, my cravings are at their strongest because I think I've screwed up and am worthless. My depression is at its worst and therefore my cravings, their most intense.

Now it's your turn to create your own cravings intensity scale. Fill in the blank worksheet completely, recording the places, times, thoughts, and feelings associated with a certain craving at every level on the scale, from 0 to 10. It may take you several days to complete the scale, since you may need to direct your awareness to your cravings before you develop a good sense of when, where, and why they arise and how to rate them. When describing your cravings and providing examples, be as specific as possible. If you need more space, use another sheet of paper. The more you know about your cravings, the more effective you'll be in trying to control them.

Cravings Intensity Worksheet

Discomfort level	Description and examples
0 No discomfort	
1	
2	
3 Mild discomfort	
4	
5	
6 Moderate discomfort	
7	
8	
9	
10 Severe discomfort	

Strategies for Overcoming Cravings

Being aware of your cravings is a great step, but it's just half the battle. You also need to resist or control them. The approach in the previous exercise can help highlight some of your trouble spots around cravings, but you still need to make the decision not to give in to them. Here are some techniques that can help you make good decisions and better manage your cravings:

Label it. Tell yourself, "This is just a craving. I've survived these cravings and feelings before without giving in to them. It's uncomfortable, maybe even intense, but it's not an emergency."

Stand firm. Tell yourself that you don't need whatever you crave. For example, "I'm not going to have a drink, even though I really want it. I truly don't need it. In the long run, it won't be worth it to give in to this craving."

Don't give yourself a choice. The difficult part about craving is struggling with what to do about it. Should you give in or not? Tell yourself, with total conviction, that you have *no choice*—that you cannot give in. Then turn to doing something else. You should find that the craving diminishes over time.

Imagine the aftermath of giving in. Think about giving in to your craving to drink, smoke, eat junk food, or buy something. How long does it take you to satisfy the craving? How long does the pleasure you get from this last? Now imagine the rest of the picture—the part of the experience you typically don't think about until it's too late. Picture yourself feeling weak and out of control. See yourself getting upset, giving up, and continuing to drink, smoke, eat junk food, or buy more and more stuff. Imagine the potential outcomes, such as liver disease, emphysema, being terribly overweight, or being bogged down in debt, and how this will make you feel worse and worse. Remind yourself of times when you've given up before and how hopeless you felt when you did.

Distance yourself from things you crave. Don't keep the things you crave in your home, workplace, or car. If you must keep something you crave nearby, perhaps unhealthy food that other family members eat, store it in an inconvenient place or somewhere you can't see it. If you're experiencing strong cravings and can't get rid of the thing you crave, remove yourself from the situation.

Drink a no-calorie or low-calorie beverage. This strategy is mostly to help with food cravings, since you can fill up on water or another low-calorie beverage instead of food. Drink something like club soda, water with lemon juice, or herbal tea and see if your craving subsides. Although this strategy is mostly aimed at food cravings, you could also try drinking something healthy to substitute for drinking alcohol or having a cigarette, or to distract you from wanting to buy something.

Relax. Stress or being in a bad mood can increase cravings. Relaxation will help with this. You can use a variety of relaxation techniques. For example, you could vividly imagine being in a favorite place, or you could take ten deep breaths and focus on your breathing, breathing deeply enough that you notice your abdomen rising and falling with each breath.

Distract yourself. Do something for a short period of time to divert your attention from the craving. You could call a friend, go for a walk, read an engaging book or article, or watch a funny video. Keep in mind that distraction is different than *avoidance*, meaning distracting yourself without awareness that you're doing so. Avoidance can be dangerous because when you aren't tuning in to what you're doing or why you've chosen to distract yourself, you may promote unhealthy behaviors, such as watching movies or TV for hours on end.

Summary

♦ Awareness is the first step in making positive, healthy decisions.

♦ Awareness can be more difficult for people with bipolar disorder because they tend to be impulsive and have difficulties with insight.

♦ Tracking your mood can help you be more aware of when you're in the best position to make better choices.

♦ Creating a cravings intensity scale can improve your awareness of your cravings, increasing your chances of resisting them.

♦ There are several techniques that can help you make better decisions when you have a craving.

Chapter 10

Finding and Keeping Support

Creating a healthy lifestyle and staying well can be much easier when you have a good support system. Having a good support system has been shown to increase well-being, and it may even help prevent depression (Sheldon and Wills 1985; Paykel 1994). Friends and family members who are supportive can provide assistance and insight in solving difficult situations and help you feel better when you have negative thoughts about yourself.

Yet relationships can be challenging. They're often the hardest things anyone works on in life. They're sometimes unpredictable, occasionally painful, and constantly a test of people's ability to regulate their emotions. For all of these reasons, they can be particularly challenging for people with bipolar disorder, in part due to false assumptions that might interfere with the ability to start and maintain relationships. So this chapter begins by examining common assumptions that people have about relationships and how to manage them. Then I'll discuss other skills that can help you to forge and maintain relationships.

Why Support Can Be Scary

There are two major fears that many people, especially those with bipolar disorder, have about relationships: fear of being hurt by others, and fear of letting others down. These fears can cause people to make many overly negative assumptions about relationships—assumptions that can make maintaining close, supportive relationships scary and difficult.

Fear of Being Hurt

You aren't alone if you're afraid that others might hurt you. Unfortunately, the people you're closest to have the potential to hurt you the most because you care about what they think. They also know what upsets you, and during a fight or conflict, they may use this against you. If you've had a close friend who let you down, or if you've had a particularly awful fight with a loved one that made you feel terrible, you know what I'm talking about. These types of interactions may make you think it's just not worth having close relationships or maintaining them. That's understandable, but it's also a thought you need to challenge. As difficult as it may feel to maintain relationships and meet new people, think about the alternative: How does it feel to be alone with your bipolar disorder?

Exercise: Coming Up with Alternative Thoughts About Relationships

To help you deal with the fear of being hurt and thoughts that relationships aren't worth the work, let's revisit a technique you learned in chapter 4: completing a thought record. You've already gotten some practice with thought records, and hopefully you've continued to use them to generate new, alternative thoughts about difficult situations. If so, you know what to do. (And as a reminder, for a downloadable version of this worksheet, visit http://www.newharbinger.com/31304; see the back of the book for more information about accessing it.) In any case, here's a quick recap:

1. Describe a difficult situation factually at the top of the worksheet—in this case, one that relates to the fear of being hurt.

2. Record negative automatic thoughts about that situation, along with the emotions associated with each thought, and rate the intensity of each emotion on a scale of 0 to 10.

3. For each automatic thought, generate at least one alternative thought that's more objective and rate the intensity of the same emotions in relation to the new thought.

Because relationships can be tricky, I've provided an example. It's for a young man who got into a fight with his mother. When reading through this example, focus on the alternative thoughts and especially how they affect the ratings of emotions. As you'll see, coming up with new thoughts made this person feel better about his relationship with his mother and reminded him of the benefits of having support.

Sample Thought Record Worksheet

Situation	Who	My mom		
	What	Talking about my schedule		
	Where	At a restaurant		
	When	Yesterday at noon		
Automatic thoughts	Emotions (0–10)	Alternative thoughts	Emotions (0–10)	
I hate that my mother tells me how I should live my life.	Embarrassment (9) Anger (5)	She suggests things for me to do because she's worried about me and wants me to feel better.	Embarrassment (5) Anger (2)	
I never should have gone to lunch. I should have just stayed at home instead.	Disappointment (8)	This lunch was difficult, but not every get-together is hard. This one was hard because my mom was trying to help me.	Disappointment (5)	
She doesn't understand my bipolar disorder.	Sadness (8) Anger (6)	My mom tries to understand my illness by reading about it, but it's difficult to understand if you haven't experienced it.	Sadness (5) Anger (2)	
No one understands my bipolar disorder.	Sadness (10) Loneliness (8)	Bipolar disorder isn't visible, so it's often misunderstood. But some people do understand, especially those who also have bipolar disorder.	Sadness (6) Loneliness (3)	
It would be better if I stayed away from people.	Sadness (10) Loneliness (10)	It can feel safer to be alone, but I never feel better when I'm alone, and I often feel worse.	Sadness (5) Loneliness (7)	
I'm destined to be alone.	Sadness (10)	If I continue to work at managing my anger and frustration with others, I can maintain my relationships and maybe meet new people.	Sadness (4)	

Thought Record Worksheet

Situation	Who	
	What	
	Where	
	When	

Automatic thoughts	Emotions (0–10)	Alternative thoughts	Emotions (0–10)

Fear of Letting Others Down

Now let's look at the other common fear in regard to relationships: that they put you at risk of letting other people down. This concern is especially relevant to people with bipolar disorder. When you're depressed or manic, you may have difficulty keeping up your end of the relationship, and you may even do or say hurtful things. During mood episodes you may cancel meetings, not show up for planned get-togethers, or not return phone calls or e-mails. And because one symptom of depression is believing that you're worthless or flawed in some way, when your mood is low you might doubt your ability to maintain relationships, much less make new friends.

But as you're now well aware, during mood episodes your thoughts often aren't accurate. They're likely to be distorted in some way. Therefore, I recommend not making any major decisions about relationships when you're experiencing a mood episode. When you're depressed, you may think you no longer want or need friends. Yet when you're either depressed or manic, your positive relationships and support systems can be enormously helpful. (In chapter 11, I'll help you make a plan for how your friends and family can support you in making healthy decisions when you aren't feeling well.)

Assertive and Effective Communication

The rest of this chapter explains the most effective communication strategy: assertiveness, which can help you manage your relationships. Assertiveness is a happy medium between passive and aggressive approaches. In *passive* communication, you don't clearly state what you want or need. This makes it difficult for others to help you. In *aggressive* communication, you may state what you want clearly, but you do so without showing consideration or respect for others. This risks angering or upsetting others and may make them unwilling or unlikely to provide support. With *assertive* communication, you state your wants and needs clearly while also respecting others. This increases the likelihood that others will understand what you need and be willing to help.

Keep in mind that you may find it much more challenging to communicate with others when you aren't feeling well. However, this is often the most important time to turn to others for support. To help you communicate more assertively, and therefore more effectively during those difficult times, I'll help you come up with a set of statements to help structure your conversations with others. But first, you need to identify what you want out of the interaction.

Knowing What You Want

Before you can practice assertiveness, skillfully asking for what you want, you first need to know *what* you want. Let's say you're feeling down and want support from a friend. Unfortunately, if you just call your friend and ask for help without getting specific, it may be hard for your friend to help you. Consider the following example.

Colleen has been feeling depressed lately. She's been sleeping fourteen hours many days, and she hardly gets out of bed because she has so little energy, motivation, and interest in life. She's started overeating—not because she's hungry, but because it occupies her time and helps her feel less empty. She's also started drinking a beer or two each night, and she fears she'll start drinking more in an attempt to cope with her low mood. She thinks her friend Amy might be able to help, so she calls her. She tells Amy that she isn't feeling well, but when Amy asks how she can help, Colleen doesn't know what to say. Colleen just wants to feel better.

Do you think Colleen will get helpful support from Amy? She might, if Amy knows her well and can help her figure out what will help her feel better. But Colleen's request would be much more effective if she first figures out what she needs and then asks for it clearly. The guidelines for setting goals can be helpful here. A request for help is much more likely to be effective if it's specific and realistic. Perhaps Amy could help Colleen stay sober some evenings by coming over and watching a movie with her. Maybe Amy and Colleen could agree to walk together a few times per week. Or maybe Amy could help Colleen go through her cupboards and get rid of all the unhealthy snack foods.

Practicing Assertiveness

Once you know what you want, you can start practicing assertiveness. To do so, you need to clearly and effectively explain why you want something. For example, imagine if Colleen were to just call Amy and ask her to come over to watch a movie. Amy may come over, but if she doesn't know Colleen wants support in not drinking that night, she may not give it a second thought when Colleen starts drinking a beer while watching the movie. Explaining the rationale—the reason Colleen wants Amy to come over—will help Amy understand what's needed and increase the likelihood of Colleen getting what she wants.

To practice communicating your requests effectively, I suggest using the following formula, which is widely recommended. Notice that all of the statements start with "I." This is very important, as no one can argue with *your* thoughts and feelings. So always stick to communicating your own thoughts, feelings, and desires, and don't make assumptions about what others think, feel, or want.

Step 1. Use an "I think" statement. This statement focuses on your understanding of what's going on and the facts of the situation. It's a clear, factual description of the situation and shouldn't include any assumptions or judgments about the situation or about other people. For Colleen, an example would be "Amy, I think I've been depressed this past week, and I've started drinking again."

Step 2. Use an "I feel" statement. This statement adds oomph to your "I think" statement, reinforcing the importance of the situation and the request you're about to make. You don't have to share your deepest, darkest emotions (and in some cases, you probably shouldn't), but you can still express an emotion that's appropriate. So Colleen might say, "I'm afraid that if I'm home alone at night, I'll just keep drinking more."

Step 3. Use an "I want" statement. This should be a very clear and specific request. Ensure that your request is realistic or doable. As discussed above, be sure to avoid using any "you" statements. (For Colleen, this could be something like "You should come over tomorrow night.") Requests using "you" statements often make people feel put upon or forced to do something. Be sure to ask for only one thing at a time, and choose something specific and realistic—something the person can do now. So, Colleen's request might be "I'd be very grateful if you could come over tomorrow evening to watch a movie with me, as this will help me stay sober."

Now put those three statements together and imagine that you're Amy. Do you understand why Colleen is calling you? Do you know how you can help her? Would you be more willing or able to help than if you'd just received a vague request for help?

Remember, no matter how good you are at asking for what you want, you still may not get it. It's important to keep this in mind so that, if you sometimes don't get what you want as you start making assertive requests, you won't think you're ineffective. You're still increasing the likelihood that you'll get what you need if you use this communication skill. The following section gives you more examples of effectively asking for or stating what you want.

Examples of Assertive Requests

To help you get a little more familiar with making assertive requests, here are a few more examples. Notice that it isn't necessary to use the precise words "I think," "I feel," or "I want." The point is to convey the intent of each.

Situation: You've been getting bored when walking by yourself, and you've noticed that your neighbor walks too. You want to talk with your neighbor about walking together.

"I think": "I've been losing motivation to walk by myself."

"I feel": "I'm worried that if I don't keep walking, I might have trouble making progress on improving my lifestyle."

"I want": "I was wondering if we could walk together one day each week."

Situation: You keep forgetting to take your medications, and your roommate is very good at remembering things.

"I think": "I have trouble remembering to do things, especially in the morning."

"I feel": "I'm afraid that if I keep forgetting to take my medications, my mood will become unstable."

"I want": "Could you stop by my room in the morning to remind me to take my medications?"

Situation: Your friend is a health nut and is constantly trying to get you to exercise and eat better.

"I think": "I seem to have a lot more trouble making healthy choices than you do."

"I feel": "I feel sad when I get reminders about things I should be doing."

"I want": "It would be really helpful for me if you could stop giving advice on what to do and instead provide more practical support. For example, when you make a salad for yourself, maybe you could make one for me too."

Situation: Your partner watches TV in bed after you'd like to go to sleep.

"I think": "I have trouble falling asleep because of the light and noise from the TV."

"I feel": "I'm worried that if I don't get good sleep, it could trigger a mood episode or worsen my symptoms."

"I want": "Could you watch your TV show in the living room?"

Situation: You live at home, and your mother tends to cook high-fat meals.

"I think": "I think that I need to be healthier, and these days I'm consuming too much fat in my meals."

"I feel": "I'm worried that if I don't eat lower-fat foods, I'll continue to have health problems."

"I want": "Could we have a salad two nights each week and make some lower-fat substitutions, such as using leaner meat or less cooking oil?"

Again, remember to avoid using "you" statements, especially any that blame others or ask them to change their thoughts or feelings. For example, steer clear of statements like "I think you should…," "I feel like you're inconsiderate (thoughtless, unkind…)," or "I want you to stop being so mean (clueless, self-centered…)." This is just dressing up aggressive communication with assertive phrasing and is likely to work out poorly. And, of course, most people don't like getting unsolicited advice or hearing negative things about themselves from others. So just talk about your own thoughts, feelings, and needs. No one can argue with what you think, feel, or want as long as you're being genuine and communicating what you really think, feel, and want.

Assertively telling others what you want or asking for help can take a lot of practice, and you may feel uncomfortable with it at first. Therefore, I suggest that you start off by making requests that aren't very difficult for you emotionally, like asking a friend to get a cup of coffee for you.

Exercise: Practicing Assertive Communication

Now it's time for you to practice assertive communication. Think of a recent situation where you wish you could have asked for help, or where you asked for help and it didn't work out well. Then try framing your request in assertive language. Then, for at least the next few weeks, use this worksheet to come up with an assertive request before asking others for help. To continue using this technique, you can just write your statements on a separate piece of paper. Or, for a downloadable version of this worksheet, visit http://www .newharbinger.com/31304. (See the back of the book for instructions on how to access it.) Continuing to practice this skill will increase the likelihood that you'll get what you need or want.

Situation (Briefly explain the facts of the situation.) _____

_____

_____

_____

"I think…" (This is what you'll say to explain the situation in your own words. Stick to the facts and avoid making assumptions.) _____

_____

_____

"I feel…" (For people you do not know very well, you can pick less intense emotions, such as "appreciate" or "concern," but do include some emotional component to emphasize why what you think and want is important to you.) _____

_____

_____

"I want…" (Be direct and specific about what you want. Ask for something that can realistically be done.) _____

_____

_____

The Broken Record Technique

The broken record technique is useful when someone isn't getting the message. It involves being persistent in stating what you want, repeating it over and over again as needed. Using short, clear statements and actually repeating them is usually most effective. Here's an example.

Jeremy: I'm going to start walking during lunch.

Leo: You'll miss what's going on in the office if you leave during lunch.

Jeremy: I think I need to get more exercise, and walking during lunch is a good way for me to do it.

Leo: Why do you feel like you need to do this all of a sudden? Who will I eat lunch with?

Jeremy: I feel that it's important for my health that I increase my activity level. I think I'll start walking during lunch tomorrow.

Leo: You're being a real jerk. You aren't understanding what I need.

Jeremy: I understand that it can be nice to eat lunch with someone, but I need to do more exercise, and I want to walk during lunch. That's a good time for me to do it.

You can see that Leo is getting more and more upset that Jeremy wants to walk during lunch. Notice that Jeremy doesn't argue back. Instead, he uses the broken record technique and even weaves in assertive communication techniques: "I think I need to get more exercise," "I feel that it's important for my health," and "I want to walk during lunch." You may also have noticed that Jeremy doesn't answer Leo's question about what he should do during lunch. Doing so would probably require using "you" statements, such as "You could eat lunch with Manuel" or "Your health isn't the greatest either; maybe you should join me on my walks." These kinds of statements give the other person ammunition for an argument; they make assumptions about the person. If you stick with your own thoughts and feelings, no one can argue with them.

Just one caution: It's usually easier to stick to your script when you're having a good day. Therefore, it probably isn't a good idea to use the broken record technique when you're very depressed or manic.

Saying No Skillfully

Learning how to say no skillfully can be very important in managing relationships. When you can't say no, it's like putting yourself on a roller-coaster ride with no brake. You'll have no control over how people treat you and what they do to you, which can make for a very bumpy and out-of-control ride. And because people with bipolar disorder tend to think negatively about themselves, their world, and their future, you may have difficulty saying no. You may want to appease others and avoid both confrontation and negative feedback. This may indeed lead to short-term gains, such as making others happy or avoiding negative interactions; but it's a passive style of interacting, and ultimately it won't serve to strengthen your relationships.

On the other hand, saying no allows you to protect yourself and be true to what you need. And bringing skill to the equation will ensure that you say no in a way that's considerate of others. This can go a long way in maintaining supportive relationships and even making new friends. There are two steps to this technique:

1. Validate the other person's needs or desires.

2. State a clear preference to not do it.

Importantly, don't say no and then give in later. This teaches people that when you say no, you don't always mean it. Therefore, they may try harder the next time to convince you not to say no. So, once you've said no, try not to change your mind. The broken record technique can be very effective here. Consider the following example.

Beth: You should split this dessert with me.

Francie: Thanks for offering to split your dessert with me, but I don't want any right now.

Beth: Come on, it's really good! You need to splurge every once in a while and have a treat. You deserve it!

Francie: It looks great, and I do agree that having dessert every so often is fine, but I don't want any dessert tonight.

Beth: Why? Are you afraid it will make you fat?

Francie: One dessert won't make anyone fat. I just don't want anything right now.

In this example, Francie says no skillfully by validating Beth and then clearly stating her refusal. Even as Beth becomes increasingly agitated about sharing her dessert, Francie chooses not to respond in a way that would give Beth something to argue about. Francie also successfully avoids using any "you" statements. As you can see, saying no effectively does require skill, but if you practice it, you will get better. To that end, the next exercise will give you some practice in saying no skillfully.

Exercise: Practicing Saying No Skillfully

In this exercise, I've provided some examples of saying no. Some are skillful; some aren't. Importantly, remember that this technique is a two-step process. In order to be skillful, a statement must validate the other person and also clearly state what you don't want to do. For each statement below, indicate whether it's validating and whether it's clear. If the statement doesn't fulfill one or both requirements, explain why. And even if a statement does fulfill both requirements, you could still explain why, just to get more familiar with this technique. Coming up with an explanation will help you with the final aspect of the exercise: writing an improved statement for each example that isn't skillful. I've done the exercise for the first few statements to give you an idea of how it works.

Situation: When deciding where to go out to eat, a woman's husband suggests the same steakhouse they went to the last time they ate out.

Sample refusal: "I can understand why you want to eat at our favorite steakhouse again, but I'd prefer not to because I'm trying to eat better."

Validating? Yes

Clear? Yes

Explanation: This statement is validating to the other person yet makes it clear that the woman won't eat at the steakhouse tonight.

Improved statement: Not needed.

Situation: A man's friend invites him to go to the park to play basketball.

Sample refusal: "I don't want to play basketball with you."

Validating? No

Clear? Yes

Explanation: There's no explanation of why this person is refusing to play basketball.

Improved statement: "Playing basketball together sounds fun, but I hurt my knee last week, so I can't play today."

Situation: A man wants to unwind and relax and asks his friend to drink a beer with him.

Sample refusal: "I know that some people find beer to be relaxing in the evening."

Validating? Yes

Clear? No

Explanation: This person isn't making it clear that she doesn't want to have a beer.

Improved statement: "I don't want a beer, but I appreciate that it's relaxing for you."

Situation 1: One of your coworkers brings a box of cupcakes to work. He eats one and then offers you one.

Sample refusal: "Please don't eat snacks near me."

Validating? _____

Clear? _____

Explanation: _____

_____

_____

Improved statement: _____

_____

Situation 2: A woman is at an outdoor music festival. A man offers her a cigarette.

Sample refusal: "I don't really like people who smoke cigarettes."

Validating? _____

Clear? _____

Explanation: _____

_____

_____

Improved statement: _____

_____

Situation 3: After a date, a woman's boyfriend says he wants to buy her an ice cream.

Sample refusal: "I don't want to eat dessert tonight, but feel free to get some ice cream for yourself."

Validating? _____

Clear? _____

Explanation: _____

_____

_____

Improved statement: _____

_____

Situation 4: A friend says she's feeling down and asks you to go to the mall with her so the two of you can do some "retail therapy" together.

Sample refusal: "I don't want to go to the mall."

Validating? _____

Clear? _____

Explanation: _____

_____

_____

Improved statement: _____

_____

Situation 5: A woman is trying to set a regular sleep schedule for herself and her partner suggests watching a movie marathon that goes late into the night.

Sample refusal: "I agree that these movies are exciting, but I don't know about watching them all night."

Validating? _____

Clear? _____

Explanation: _____

_____

_____

Improved statement: _____

_____

How did that go? In case you want to double-check your answers, they are as follows: (1) no, no; (2) no, no; (3) yes, yes; (4) no, yes; (5) yes, no.

As a reminder, when saying no, you don't want to argue or offer excessive justification for your position. Stick to the two key steps: validating and declining. Don't add anything extra. Be clear and to the point. This is the most effective strategy when saying no because it doesn't give the other person anything to use against you. Remember, no one can argue with *your* thoughts and feelings.

Summary

- Social support is a very important part of creating a healthy lifestyle.

- Using a thought record can help you overcome your fears and assumptions about relationships.

- Learning techniques for communicating more effectively can help you maintain your current relationships and make it easier to forge new relationships.

- Being assertive involves clearly and respectfully asking for what you want and expressing why it's important to you, using a script of "I think…," "I feel…," and "I want…"

- The broken record technique can be helpful when someone isn't getting the message.

- Saying no skillfully is an important part of maintaining relationships.

- There's no guarantee that using effective communication skills will get you what you want, but it will increase the likelihood.

Chapter 11

Creating a Wellness Plan

This final chapter focuses on putting together everything you've learned in this book to create a personalized wellness plan. This plan, which you'll develop with support from others, such as family members, friends, and health care professionals, will help you continue down the path of creating a healthier lifestyle. To help you draft the best possible plan, I'll start by helping you assess your areas of strength and weakness. That way your plan can help you capitalize on your strengths and build up areas of weakness. Then I'll guide you through creating a plan that is—you guessed it!—specific and realistic. Of course, your work doesn't stop there. Once you have a plan, you need to follow it to the best of your ability, rewarding yourself for your successes and modifying the plan as needed. So let's get started!

Determining Your Areas of Strength and Weakness

Before you can create any plan, you have to know the starting point. In this section, I'll help you identify both the strengths and the weaknesses you bring to creating and maintaining a healthy lifestyle. Everyone has things they're good at (strengths), as well as areas they could improve upon (weaknesses). In chapter 2, you started identifying some goals for creating a healthier lifestyle, with a focus on setting achievable goals. That may have helped you think about which kinds of changes are easier for you and which are harder.

Since chapter 2, we've covered a lot more ground, with lengthy discussions of many aspects of living a more healthy lifestyle, especially eating better, getting more active, and getting good sleep. The next two exercises will help you identify your areas of strength and weakness in these and other aspects of your lifestyle.

Exercise: Identifying Your Strengths

Take some time to really think about the things you're currently doing well. Don't sell yourself short. Everyone has strengths, and you're no exception. If you can't think of anything you're doing well, review the material on awareness in chapter 9, because chances are you simply aren't aware that you're doing well in certain areas.

The following form lists some common lifestyle changes that contribute to a healthier lifestyle. Which of these are relatively easy for you? Read through the list and check those that are easier, then use the empty rows to fill in other strengths not listed here.

Also take a moment to describe why each of these changes is relatively easy for you. Here are some examples of what you might write in the right-hand column for why some of the healthy habits listed below are easy for you to adopt.

- If you're successful at drinking plenty of water because there's a water cooler near your desk, write that in the right-hand column. And if drinking lots of water helps you avoid or resist cravings, that's a bonus. Write that down too.

- If you've found it easy to walk regularly because a neighbor has been joining you for walks, record that in the right-hand column.

- If you've been successful in stretching because you're sore from your new walking routine, and stretching feels good, write it down!

- If you're successful in not using alcohol and other substances because you've experienced how much better you feel when you don't use them, or because you know it's dangerous to mix them with your bipolar medications, write that in the right-hand column.

Assessing Your Strengths

✔	Healthy habits that are easy for you to adopt	Why is this habit easy?
	Eating more fruits and vegetables	
	Eating reasonable portion sizes	
	Limiting or forgoing sweets	
	Drinking plenty of water	
	Doing moderate-intensity exercise	
	Doing occasional strength training	
	Stretching	
	Keeping a good sleep schedule	
	Not using drugs or alcohol	
	Taking my bipolar medications	

✔	Healthy habits that are easy for you to adopt	Why is this habit easy?

Exercise: Identifying Your Areas for Improvement

Now let's go through a similar process for your weaknesses—but let's call those "areas for improvement" instead, to keep a positive perspective. Which healthy habits are hardest for you to adopt? Be honest here and remember that the purpose is to help you create a healthier lifestyle, not beat yourself up.

This time, the following worksheet lists some common habits that keep people from adopting a healthier lifestyle. Read through the list and check any habits that you're having a hard time breaking, then use the empty rows to fill in other areas for improvement not listed here. Of course, the flipside of anything in the previous list of strengths could be a weakness—for example, not eating many fruits and vegetables, not eating reasonable portion sizes, and so on. Also take a moment to describe, in the right-hand column, why each of these habits is hard for you to break. Here are a few examples.

- If you have trouble exercising regularly because you think it won't really help you lose weight, write that in the right-hand column.

- If you have trouble sleeping and tend to stay up late because you have racing thoughts when you go to bed at night, write that down.

- If you smoke cigarettes because it seems to soothe your mood or calm your mind, write that in the right-hand column.

- If you tend to isolate yourself a lot because you often feel depressed, which reduces your motivation and makes you feel like no one would want to spend time with you anyway, write it down.

Assessing Your Areas for Improvement

✔	Unhealthy habits that are hard for you to break	Why is it hard to break this habit?
	Eating too much junk food or unhealthy high-fat foods	
	Overeating	
	Eating out a lot	
	Not exercising regularly	
	Going to bed very late or keeping an erratic sleep schedule	
	Smoking cigarettes	
	Using alcohol or other substances	
	Buying too many new things	
	Isolating and not seeing friends and family	
	Not seeing a therapist or psychiatrist regularly	

✔	Unhealthy habits that are hard for you to break	Why is it hard to break this habit?

Exercise: Using Your Strengths and Areas for Improvement to Identify Your Wellness Goals

In the preceding two exercises, you identified the healthy habits that are easiest for you to follow and why, and then identified your areas for improvement and why you have difficulty breaking certain habits. Now you'll use this work to create a set of goals for your wellness plan. To do so, you'll build on your strengths and find ways to set yourself up for success in areas that need improvement. In terms of strengths, say you just happen to like the taste of fruit, so it's easy for you to eat plenty of it; or you enjoy walking, so you're successful at being active when it takes this form. Be sure to include your most healthy habits on your wellness plan as goals you'd like to continue to meet.

It may be a bit more challenging to identify goals related to areas that need improvement. For example, perhaps you tend to buy too many new things. What kind of wellness goal might you set to help reduce your spending? You have to figure out what will work for you, but possibilities include giving up your credit cards or setting a strict budget for yourself. Another possibility is that your strengths will give you some insights into how you might work with your areas for improvement. Say you identified "Eating too much junk food" as an area for improvement, and in the right-hand column you wrote that this habit is hard to break because you have strong food cravings when you're depressed or bored. If, under strengths, you noted that it's easy for you to eat fruit because you love the flavors of fruits, you might begin to choose fruits, rather than junk food, when cravings hit.

Keeping in mind the advice in chapter 2 to not set too many goals at once, now choose three strengths to build upon in your wellness plan and three areas for improvement and write them in the following worksheet. Then set a specific wellness goal for each. If you aren't sure about the best goals to set for yourself, don't worry. Look at them as a starting point. You can always modify them if they don't work well for you.

To identify suitable goals, you can also review earlier chapters, looking to chapters 3 and 4 for guidance on potential goals related to nutrition and healthy eating, chapters 5 and 6 for ideas about goals to increase your activity level, and chapter 8 for potential goals related to sleep. And if you have trouble with motivation, revisit chapter 7 and consider using rewards to increase your motivation to stick with your goals.

To give you an idea of how this works, I've provided a sample worksheet, followed by a blank version for your use.

Wellness Goals

Strengths to build upon	Wellness goals
1. Stretching	Stretch for 5 to 10 minutes before each walk with my neighbor, and make sure I stretch at least three days per week.
2. Drinking water	Visit the water cooler at least once every hour while at work.
3. Walking	Continue to walk four days a week, but increase my weekly distance by 0.5 mile each week.

Areas to improve upon	Wellness goals
1. Sleep	Set a target bedtime of midnight, and time to get out of bed at 9 a.m. Start my bedtime routine at 11 p.m. to create a wind-down time before bed.
2. Smoking	Smoke one less cigarette a day this week. If I have cravings, consider sucking on a hard candy or having a piece of gum, or distracting myself.
3. Friends and social support	Attend a Depression and Bipolar Support Alliance meeting one day per week, and start volunteering as a way to meet more people.

Wellness Goals

Strengths to build upon	Wellness goals
1.	
2.	
3.	

Areas to improve upon	Wellness goals
1.	
2.	
3.	

Creating Your Wellness Plan

Now that you've identified your strengths, weaknesses, and a few wellness goals based on them, you can put all of this together to create your wellness plan. You might think of this plan as a contract. It's an agreement between your healthy self (when you want to make positive lifestyle changes) and your unhealthy self (when you don't want to make such changes). This commitment is important because when you're experiencing bipolar symptoms or otherwise aren't feeling well, you may not think you need to stick to your plan, or you may lack motivation to do so. Creating a contract with yourself in advance of those times will remind you that you promised yourself (and your friends, family, and care providers) that you'd do these things, even when you're feeling unwell. For this reason, you need to sign your wellness plan once you've finalized it.

I've provided a blank worksheet that you can use to document your wellness plan. Since you'll probably want to create new plans as you're ready to work toward new goals, or as your life changes, a downloadable version of the worksheet is available at http://www .newharbinger.com/31304. (See the back of the book for instructions on how to access it.) The blank version appears a bit later in the chapter. In the sections that follow, I'll guide you through each part of the worksheet and provide examples of each:

1. Identifying your support team

2. Identifying early signs of a lapse

3. Identifying the signs of a more severe lapse

4. Taking action to create a healthier lifestyle by adhering to your wellness plan

5. Signing your plan to indicate your commitment to following it

You can either create your plan in the blank worksheet as you read through each section below, or read all of the sections to get an overview of the process and then fill in the worksheet—whichever works best for you. And either way, you may want to seek help or advice from your support team before finalizing your plan. Their feedback will probably prove very helpful in creating a workable plan. Also, bear in mind that creating your plan is a detailed and potentially lengthy task. Take your time and be thoughtful, and be sure to set specific, realistic goals for yourself. You may want to work on it over the course of a few days or a week. In the end, it will be worth the time and effort. You're establishing a structure that will help you adopt a healthier lifestyle and experience greater well-being.

Section 1. Identifying Your Support Team

Section 1 of the worksheet provides a place to record the members of your support team. Identify trusted people—at least three, preferably five—that you can call on when you need help. These people may be friends, family members, care providers, other professionals, spiritual leaders, or anyone else who can either help you with specific goals or provide more general support and encouragement in following through with your plan. Each of these people will sign your wellness plan and receive a copy of it. Be sure to record contact information for each person when filling out this section of the plan.

1. My Support Team		
Name	**Role or relationship**	**Contact information**
My mom	My mom	phone number, address, or e-mail
Bill	My brother	phone number, address, or e-mail
Anita	My friend/neighbor	phone number, address, or e-mail
Dr. Milton	My therapist	phone number, address, or e-mail
Dr. Ham	My psychiatrist	phone number, address, or e-mail
Reverend Walters	My spiritual mentor	phone number, address, or e-mail

Section 2. Identifying Early Signs of a Lapse

The next step in creating your wellness plan is to identify the early signs that you may be starting to lapse into old, unhealthy habits—or developing new ones. Give some thought to what the early warning signs would be for you, then record your top five signs in the left-hand column of section 2 of your wellness plan. It's crucial to identify early and more subtle signs of a lapse, since it's usually easier to take corrective action just as you're beginning to slip.

In the right-hand column, list how you think slipping back into each unhealthy habit will affect your mood or other areas of your life. Of course, if you actually lapse in a certain area, it may affect you differently than you anticipated. Make your best guess now, and if you later discover it isn't correct, note what actually happens. Either way, this will help you to monitor both your lifestyle and your mood episodes, as well as the connections between them. Lifestyle changes can often cause changes in your bipolar symptoms, and vice versa. For example, you may notice that you have a bigger appetite or tend to crave pizza just before becoming depressed. By identifying this important connection between unhealthy habits and your mood, you'll be in a better position to get back on track with a healthier lifestyle and also prevent your depression from getting worse. Finally, be sure to review both this section and section 3 with your support team so they can help you monitor and manage your wellness.

2. Identifying Early Signs of a Lapse	
Change in healthy habit	**How this change will affect you**
I begin to walk less frequently with my neighbor.	I feel sadder and less energetic when I walk less often.
I eat more sweets at night to fill myself up before bed.	I feel down on myself, especially because I don't even really like sweets.
I start drinking more coffee at work and stop drinking water.	I feel even more tired about an hour after drinking a cup of coffee and want more. It never really makes me feel better or more energetic.
I start watching late night movies.	I stay up later and feel more tired in the morning.
I stop going to my weekly Depression and Bipolar Support Alliance meeting.	I feel less connected with other people and more alone.

Section 3. Identifying the Signs of a More Severe Lapse

It's also a good idea to list some signs of a more severe lapse. Think of these as red alerts, signaling that it's extremely important to get back on track. These are also signals to reach out for help. So give some thought to what the warning signs of a more severe lapse would be for you, then record your top five signs in the left-hand column of section 3 of the worksheet, as shown in the example below.

Then, in the right-hand column, list how you think slipping back into each unhealthy habit will affect your mood or other areas of your life. Again, if you actually lapse in a certain area, it may affect you differently than you anticipated. Make your best guess now, and if you later discover it isn't correct, note what actually happens.

3. Identifying the Signs of a More Severe Lapse	
Change in healthy habit	**How this change will affect you**
I start eating unhealthy afternoon snacks, like chips or a candy bar.	*I start thinking that I'll get fat, and then I feel sad.*
I start smoking more cigarettes again.	*I get angry with myself because I know smoking isn't good for me. It does help ease my anxiety and agitation, but that's very short-lived.*
I no longer cook meals.	*I begin to eat out more often, making it more difficult to choose healthy options.*
I stop taking some of my bipolar medications because I think they don't matter or make a difference.	*My mood starts to become more unstable, and I get more depressed and also more agitated.*
I stop returning phone calls from friends and family.	*I start spending more time alone and feel lonely.*

Section 4. Taking Action to Create a Healthier Lifestyle

For section 4 of the worksheet, in the "Things to do" column fill in the wellness goals you identified earlier in this chapter. These specific, realistic goals will set the stage for you to take action to create a healthier lifestyle. The goals you record in this section of your plan form the heart of your plan. All of the other elements of the plan are designed to help you keep these goals in mind.

As you'll see, the worksheet includes a number of basic items that are central to a healthy lifestyle for people with bipolar disorder. Those I've included are the ones my clients most often find important. However, the blank version also has space for you to record the wellness goals you identified earlier in the chapter. In the right-hand column, note who could provide support for each goal. For example, perhaps you're willing to have your mom help you with creating your daily schedule, but you'd prefer to have a friend remind you about the importance of exercising or eating right. Knowing who can help you and when is a very important part of creating your wellness plan, so be sure to give this some careful thought.

4. Taking Action to Create a Healthier Lifestyle		
✔	Things to do	Who can provide support?
✔	Contact a doctor, therapist, or counselor: *Dr. Milton or Dr. Ham.*	*My mom*
✔	Contact a support person: *My mom.*	*Bill*
	Eat more nutritiously.	
✔	Eat less, or eat more reasonable portions.	*Anita, Rev. Walters*
✔	Increase my activity level on a daily basis.	*Anita*
✔	Evaluate my thinking and use cognitive restructuring.	*Dr. Ham*
✔	Reward myself for making healthy choices.	*Rev. Walters*
✔	Maintain a regular sleep schedule.	*Dr. Milton, Anita*
✔	Maintain a regular schedule of activities.	*My mom, Bill*
✔	Make sure I take my medications.	*My mom*
	Reduce or quit drinking alcohol.	
✔	Reduce or quit smoking cigarettes.	*Bill*
✔	Reduce or quit consuming caffeine.	*Anita*

✔	Work on strategies for overcoming my cravings.	*Anita, my mom*
✔	Break larger tasks into smaller ones in order to complete them.	*Anita*
✔	Do a positive activity.	*My mom*
✔	Other: *Schedule 1 hour of wind-down time from 11 p.m. to midnight.*	*My mom*
✔	Other: *Walk with Anita three days per week.*	*Anita*
✔	Other: *Stretch for at least ten minutes before each walk.*	*Anita*
✔	Other: *Smoke one less cigarette than usual each day this week.*	*Bill*
✔	Other: *Drink at least 2 quarts of water each day.*	*My mom*
✔	Other: *Attend a Depression and Bipolar Support Alliance meeting.*	*Rev. Walters*

Section 5. Signing Your Plan

The final step in creating your wellness plan is to sign and date it, documenting your commitment to following your plan. Also ask each member of your support team to read the plan and sign this section, affirming their agreement to help you adhere to your plan. Remember, you're making a contract with yourself, as well as with your support team, to do the things you've outlined in section 4 to help you live a healthier lifestyle. Section 5 of your plan will also serve as a reminder that you do have support. Each person who signs the plan should receive a copy of it and keep it in an easily accessible place.

Exercise: Creating Your Wellness Plan

If you haven't already begun to fill out the Wellness Plan Worksheet, now's the time. The blank form for your use is provided. (As a reminder, a downloadable version of this worksheet is available at http://www.newharbinger.com/31304.)

Wellness Plan Worksheet

1. My Support Team		
Name	Role or relationship	Contact information

2. Identifying Early Signs of a Lapse

Change in healthy habit	How this change will affect you

3. Identifying Signs of a More Severe Lapse

Change in healthy habit	How this change will affect you

4. Taking Action to Create a Healthier Lifestyle		
✔	Things to do	Who can provide support?
	Contact a doctor, therapist, or counselor (specify who):	
	Contact a support person (specify who):	
	Eat more nutritiously.	
	Eat less, or eat more reasonable portions.	
	Increase my activity level on a daily basis.	
	Evaluate my thinking and use cognitive restructuring.	
	Reward myself for making healthy choices.	
	Maintain a regular sleep schedule.	
	Maintain a regular schedule of activities.	
	Make sure I take my medications.	
	Reduce or quit drinking alcohol.	
	Reduce or quit smoking cigarettes.	
	Reduce or quit consuming caffeine.	
	Work on strategies for overcoming my cravings.	
	Break larger tasks into smaller ones in order to complete them.	
	Do a positive activity.	
	Other:	
	Other:	
	Other:.	
	Other:	
	Other:	

5. Signatures	
_____	_____
Your signature	Date
_____	_____
Support person's signature	Date
_____	_____
Support person's signature	Date
_____	_____
Support person's signature	Date

Adapted from Gary Sachs, *Managing Bipolar Affective Disorder* (London: Science Press, 2004). Copyright © 2004 Gary Sachs. All rights reserved. Used here with permission.

Using Your Wellness Plan

Of course, the most important part of creating a wellness plan is to actually use it. So review it often and assess whether you're basically following the plan and working toward the goals you've set for yourself. You might even want to keep a copy of your plan with you as a reminder of what you've committed to doing. Sections 2 and 3, which identify your early and more severe signs of lapses are especially important to review often so you'll notice whether you're slipping and can take whatever action is needed to follow your plan.

It's important that you review and follow your wellness plan when you're feeling well and not experiencing many bipolar symptoms, for two reasons: First, you'll probably find it easier to adhere to your plan when you're feeling well. And second, practicing your new lifestyle habits when you're well will make it easier for you to stick with them when you're experiencing a mood episode or other symptoms. This is a good thing, because the most important time to follow your wellness plan is when you're experiencing bipolar symptoms. It will be harder to maintain your healthy habits then, but doing so will help you avoid many negative outcomes, including damaging your relationships, developing problems at work, gaining too much weight, or making decisions you might regret later. Your wellness plan is intended to keep you as healthy as possible, even—and especially—when you aren't feeling well.

Modifying Your Plan

One final but very important point: If your wellness plan doesn't help you adhere to a healthy lifestyle, you need to modify it. So review it from time to time and, perhaps with the input of your support team, modify what isn't working. For example, you may identify additional skills that would be helpful and want to add them to your plan. Or perhaps you'll discover that some skills on your plan are no longer relevant, aren't really helping you, or just aren't feasible, especially when you aren't feeling well. Remove these skills or goals from your plan and substitute new ones that are more helpful, relevant, or achievable. Remember, your wellness plan should be realistic: feasible and achievable for you. If it isn't, you need to modify it.

On the other hand, if you're able to follow your plan most or all of the time, it might be a good idea to set the bar a little higher. In this case, replace some of the goals you've achieved or consider replacing some of the easier skills with others that are a bit more of a stretch for you. And, of course, life is ever changing. Sometimes you'll need to revise your plan to adjust to new circumstances or challenges.

Another consideration is your support team. As you change your plan and specific goals, you may find that you need to change your support team because other people can better support you in following your new plan. You may also decide that you need to change members of your support team for other reasons, perhaps because of life changes (yours or others') or because you determine that a different person may be more helpful in certain areas.

You may need to modify your wellness plan several times before you come up with something that really works for you, especially as you first start using this approach. That's fine. You don't need to create a perfect plan, or even succeed in following your plan all the time; you just need to identify healthy lifestyle changes that are important for you and strategies that can help you achieve them. Throughout, remember that friends, family members, care providers, and other members of your support team can be very helpful in creating a wellness plan that works for you.

Each time you create a new plan, use a fresh worksheet to document it, and be sure that you and all of the members of your support team sign off on it. Remember, it's a contract. If you treat it as such, you'll be well on the way to greater health and wellness. I wish you all the best!

Summary

♦ A wellness plan is a contract between yourself when you're feeling well and yourself when you aren't well.

♦ A wellness plan will help you to adhere to healthy lifestyle goals, especially when you aren't feeling well.

♦ A wellness plan is most likely to be helpful if you incorporate input from others who know you well.

♦ You have to follow your wellness plan for it to be effective, so it needs to be feasible.

♦ A wellness plan that isn't feasible or otherwise isn't working must be modified.

References

Alloy, L. B., L. Y. Abramson, P. D. Walshaw, and A. M. Neerren. 2006. "Cognitive Vulnerability to Unipolar and Bipolar Mood Disorders." *Journal of Social and Clinical Psychology* 25(7): 726–754.

American College of Sports Medicine. 2005. *ACSM's Guidelines for Exercise Testing and Prescription*. Baltimore: Lippincott, Williams, and Wilkins.

American Psychiatric Association. 2013. *Diagnostic and Statistical Manual of Mental Disorders*, 5th edition. Washington, DC: Author.

Angst, F., H. H. Stassen, P. J. Clayton, and J. Angst. 2002. "Mortality of Patients with Mood Disorders: Follow-up Over 34–38 Years." *Journal of Affective Disorders* 68(2–3): 167–181.

Arroll, B., and R. Beaglehole. 1992. "Does Physical Activity Lower Blood Pressure: A Critical Review of the Clinical Trials." *Journal of Clinical Epidemiology* 45(5): 439–565.

Babyak, M., J. A. Blumenthal, S. Herman, P. Khatri, M. Doraiswamy, K. Moore, W. E. Craighead, T. T. Baldewicz, and K. R. Krishnan. 2000. "Exercise Treatment for Major Depression: Maintenance of Therapeutic Benefit at 10 Months." *Psychosomatic Medicine* 62(5): 633–638.

Balanzá-Martínez, V., G. R. Fries, G. D. Colpo, P. P. Silveira, A. K. Portella, R. Tabarés-Seisdedos, and F. Kapczinski. 2011. "Therapeutic Use of Omega-3 Fatty Acids in Bipolar Disorder." *Expert Review of Neurotherapeutics* 11(7): 1029–1047.

Beck, A. T., A. J. Rush, B. F. Saw, and G. Emery. 1979. *Cognitive Therapy of Depression*. New York: Guilford.

Beck, J. S. 2011. *Cognitive Behavior Therapy, Second Edition: Basics and Beyond*. New York: Guilford.

Binder, D. K., and H. E. Scharfman. 2004. "Brain-Derived Neurotrophic Factor." *Growth Factors* 22(3): 123–131.

Blumenthal, J. A., M. A. Babyak, K. A. Moore, W. E. Craighead, S. Herman, P. Khatri, et al. 1999. "Effects of Exercise Training on Older Patients with Major Depression." *Archives of Internal Medicine* 159(19): 2349–2356.

Brownell, K. D. 2000. *The LEARN Program for Weight Management 2000.* Euless, TX: American Health Publishing Company.

Buoli, M., A. Caldiroli, E. Caletti, E. Zugno, and A. C. Altamura. 2014. "The Impact of Mood Episodes and Duration of Illness on Cognition in Bipolar Disorder." *Comprehensive Psychiatry* 55(7): 1561–1566.

Cappuccio, F. P., L. D'Elia, P. Strazzullo, and M. A. Miller. 2010. "Sleep Duration and All-Cause Mortality: A Systematic Review and Meta-Analysis of Prospective Studies." *Sleep* 35(5): 585–592.

Cassidy, F., E. P. Ahearn, and B. J. Carroll. 2001. "Substance Abuse in Bipolar Disorder." *Bipolar Disorders* 3(4): 181–188.

Diabetes Prevention Program Research Group. 1999. "The Diabetes Prevention Program: Design and Methods for a Clinical Trial in the Prevention of Type 2 Diabetes." *Diabetes Care* 22(4): 623–634.

Duman, R. S. 2005. "Neurotrophic Factors and Regulation of Mood: Role of Exercise, Diet, and Metabolism." *Neurobiology of Aging* 26(suppl 1): 88–93.

Edenfield, T. M. 2008. "Exercise and Mood: Exploring the Role of Exercise in Regulating Stress Reactivity in Bipolar Disorder." *Dissertation Abstracts International: Section B: The Sciences and Engineering* 68(8–B): 5566.

Ernst, C., A. K. Olson, J. P. Pinel, R. W. Lam, and B. R. Christie. 2006. "Antidepressant Effects of Exercise: Evidence for an Adult-Neurogensis Hypothesis?" *Journal of Psychiatry Neuroscience* 31(2): 84–91.

Ettinger, W. H., R. Burns, S. P. Messier, W. Applegate, J. Rejeski, T. Morgan, S. Shumaker, M. J. Berry, M. O'Toole, J. Monu, and T. Craven. 1997. "A Randomized Trial Comparing Aerobic Exercise and Resistance Exercise with a Health Education Program in Older Adults with Knee Osteoarthritis: The Fitness Arthritis and Seniors Trial (FAST)." *JAMA* 277(1): 25–31.

Evans, S., R. Newton, and S. Higgins. 2005. "Nutritional Intervention to Prevent Weight Gain in Patients Commenced on Olanzapine: A Randomized Controlled Trial." *Australian and New Zealand Journal of Psychiatry* 39(6): 479–486.

Fagiolini, A., K. N. Chengappa, I. Soreca, and J. Chang. 2008. "Bipolar Disorder and the Metabolic Syndrome: Causal Factors, Psychiatric Outcomes and Economic Burden." *CNS Drugs* 22(8): 655–669.

Fong, A. J., S. De Jesus, S. R. Bray, and H. Prapavessis. 2014. "Effect of Exercise on Cigarette Cravings and Ad Libitum Smoking Following Concurrent Stressors." *Addictive Behaviors* 39(10): 1516–1521.

Garber, C. E., B. Blissmer, M. R. Deschenes, B. A. Franklin, M. J. Lamonte, I. M. Lee, D. C. Nieman, D. P. Swain, and American College of Sports Medicine. 2011. "American College of Sports Medicine Position Stand. Quantity and Quality of Exercise for Developing and Maintaining Cardiorespiratory, Musculoskeletal, and Neuromotor Fitness in Apparently Healthy Adults: Guidance for Prescribing Exercise." *Medicine and Science in Sports and Exercise* 43(7): 1334–1359.

Goldapple, K., Z. Segal, C. Garson, M. Lau, P. Bieling, S. Kennedy, and H. Mayberg. 2004. "Modulation of Cortical-Limbic Pathways in Major Depression: Treatment-Specific Effects of Cognitive Behavior Therapy." *Archives of General Psychiatry* 61(1): 34–41.

Grant, B. F., F. S. Stinson, D. S. Hasin, D. A. Dawson, S. P. Chou, W. J. Ruan, and B. Huang. 2006. "Prevalence, Correlates, and Comorbidity of Bipolar I Disorder and Axis I and II Disorders: Results from the National Epidemiologic Survey on Alcohol and Related Conditions." *Journal of Clinical Psychiatry* 66(10): 1205–1215.

Greenberger, D., and C. A. Padesky. 1995. *Mind Over Mood: Change How You Feel by Changing the Way You Think.* New York: Guilford.

Gruber, J., A. G. Harvey, P. W. Wang, J. O. Brooks III, M. E. Thase, G. S. Sachs, and T. A. Ketter. 2009. "Sleep Functioning in Relation to Mood, Function, and Quality of Life at Entry to the Systematic Treatment Enhancement Program for Bipolar Disorder (STEP-BD)." *Journal of Affective Disorders* 114(1–3): 41–49.

Harvey, A. G. 2008. "Sleep and Circadian Rhythms in Bipolar Disorder: Seeking Synchrony, Harmony, and Regulation." *American Journal of Psychiatry* 165(7): 820–829.

Harvey, A. G., D. A. Schmidt, A. Scarnà, C. N. Semler, and G. M. Goodwin. 2005. "Sleep-Related Functioning in Euthymic Patients with Bipolar Disorder, Patients with Insomnia, and Subjects with Sleep Problems." *American Journal of Psychiatry* 162(1): 50–57.

Haslam, D. W., and W. P. James. 2005. "Obesity." *Lancet* 366(9492): 1197–1209.

Heffner, J. L., R. M. Anthenelli, C. M. Adler, S. M. Strakowski, J. Beavers, and M. P. DelBello. 2013. "Prevalence and Correlates of Heavy Smoking and Nicotine Dependence in Adolescents with Bipolar and Cannabis Use Disorders." *Psychiatry Research* 210(3): 857–862.

Hepworth, R., K. Mogg, C. Brignell, and B. P. Bradley. 2010. "Negative Mood Increases Selective Attention to Food Cues and Subjective Appetite." *Appetite* 54(1): 134–142.

Hirschfeld, R. M., and L. A. Vornik. 2005. "Bipolar Disorder: Costs and Comorbidity." *American Journal of Managed Care* 11(3 suppl): S85–S90.

Hooper, L., C. D. Summerbell, R. Thompson, D. Sills, F. G. Roberts, H. Moore, and G. Davey Smith. 2011. "Reduced or Modified Dietary Fat for Preventing Cardiovascular Disease." *Cochrane Database of Systematic Reviews* July 6(7): CD002137.

Hu, F. B., R. J. Sigal, J. W. Rich-Edwards, G. A. Colditz, C. G. Solomon, W. C. Willett, F. E. Speizer, and J. E. Manson. 1999. "Walking Compared with Vigorous Physical Activity and Risk of Type 2 Diabetes in Women." *JAMA* 282(15): 1433–1439.

Huxley, N. A., S. V. Parikh, and R. J. Baldessarini. 2000. "Effectiveness of Psychosocial Treatments in Bipolar Disorder: State of the Evidence." *Harvard Review of Psychiatry* 8(3): 126–140.

Ingvar, D. H. 1985. "'Memory of the Future': An Essay on the Temporal Organization of Conscious Awareness." *Human Neurobiology* 4(3): 127–136.

Institute of Medicine. 2014. *Dietary Reference Intakes for Water, Potassium, Sodium, Chloride, and Sulfate.* Washington, DC: National Academies.

Johnson, S. L., and J. E. Roberts. 1995. "Life Events and Bipolar Disorder: Implications from Biological Theories." *Psychological Bulletin* 117(3): 434–449.

Jones, S. H., D. J. Hare, and K. Evershed. 2005. "Actigraphic Assessment of Circadian Activity and Sleep Patterns in Bipolar Disorder." *Bipolar Disorders* 7(2): 176–186.

Keitner, G. I., D. A. Solomon, C. E. Ryan, I. W. Miller, A. Mallinger, D. J. Kupfer, and E. Frank. 1996. "Prodromal and Residual Symptoms in Bipolar I Disorder." *Comprehensive Psychiatry* 37(5): 362–367.

Kilbourne, A. M., E. P. Post, A. Nossek, L. Drill, S. Cooley, and M. S. Bauer. 2008. "Improving Medical and Psychiatric Outcomes Among Individuals with Bipolar Disorder: A Randomized Controlled Trial." *Psychiatry Services* 59(7): 760–768.

Kilbourne, A. M., D. L. Rofey, J. F. McCarthy, E. Post, D. Welsh, and F. C. Blow. 2007. "Nutrition and Exercise Behavior Among Patients with Bipolar Disorder." *Bipolar Disorders* 9(5): 443–452.

Knowler, W. C., E. Barrett-Connor, S. E. Fowler, R. F. Hamman, J. M. Lachin, E. A. Walker, D. M. Nathan, and Diabetes Prevention Program Research Group. 2002. "Reduction in the Incidence of Type 2 Diabetes with Lifestyle Intervention or Metformin." *New England Journal of Medicine* 346(6): 393–403.

Kupfer, D. J. 2005. "The Increasing Medical Burden in Bipolar Disorder." *JAMA* 293(20): 2528–2530.

Linehan, M. 1993. *Cognitive-Behavioral Treatment of Borderline Personality Disorder.* New York: Guilford.

Lu, B. 2003. "BDNF and Activity-Dependent Synaptic Modulation." *Learning and Memory* 10(2): 86–98.

Malkoff-Schwartz, S., E. Frank, B. Anderson, J. T. Sherrill, L. Siegel, D. Patterson, and D. J. Kupfer. 1998. "Stressful Life Events and Social Rhythm Disruption in the Onset of Manic and Depressive Bipolar Episodes: A Preliminary Investigation." *Archives of General Psychiatry* 55(8): 702–707.

McKay, M., J. Wood., and J. Brantley. 2007. *The Dialectical Behavior Therapy Skills Workbook: Practical DBT Exercises for Learning Mindfulness, Interpersonal Effectiveness, Emotion Regulation, and Distress Tolerance.* Oakland, CA: New Harbinger.

Mischoulon, D., and M. F. Raab. 2007. "The Role of Folate in Depression and Dementia." *Journal of Clinical Psychiatry* 68(suppl 10): 28–33.

National Center for Health Statistics. 2013. *Health, United States, 2012: With Special Feature on Emergency Care.* Hyattsville, MD: Author.

Ng, F., S. Dodd, and M. Berk. 2007. "The Effects of Physical Activity in the Acute Treatment of Bipolar Disorder: A Pilot Study." *Journal of Affective Disorders* 101(1–3): 259–262.

Ng, T. H., K. F. Chung, F. Y. Ho, W. F. Yeung, K. P. Yung, and T. H. Lam. 2014. "Sleep-Wake Disturbance in Interepisode Bipolar Disorder and High-Risk Individuals: A Systematic Review and Meta-Analysis." *Sleep Medicine Reviews*. [Epub ahead of print.]

Ostacher, M. J., A. A. Nierenberg, R. H. Perlis, P. Eidelman, D. J. Borrelli, T. B. Tran, G. Marzilli Ericson, R. D. Weiss, and G. S. Sachs. 2006. "The Relationship Between Smoking and Suicidal Behavior, Comorbidity, and Course of Illness in Bipolar Disorder." *Journal of Clinical Psychiatry* 67(12): 1907–1911.

Park, D. H., J. Yu, and S. H. Ryu. 2006. "Alcohol and Sleep." *Sleep Medicine and Psychophysiology* 13(1): 5–10.

Paykel, E. S. 1994. "Life Events, Social Support, and Depression." *Acta Psychiatrica Scandinavica* 89(suppl 377): 50–58.

Plante, D. T., and J. W. Winkelman. 2008. "Sleep Disturbance in Bipolar Disorder: Therapeutic Implications." *American Journal of Psychiatry* 165(7): 830–843.

Popkin, B. M., K. E. D'Anci, and I. H. Rosenberg. 2010. "Water, Hydration, and Health." *Nutrition Reviews* 68(8): 439–458.

Prochaska, J. O., J. C. Norcross, and C. C. DiClemente. 1994. *Changing for Good: A Revolutionary Six-Stage Program for Overcoming Bad Habits and Moving Your Life Positively Forward*. New York: Avon.

Ravindran, A. V., and T. L. da Silva. 2013. "Complementary and Alternative Therapies as Add-On to Pharmacotherapy for Mood and Anxiety Disorders: A Systematic Review." *Journal of Affective Disorders* 150(3): 707–719.

Rice, B. H., E. E. Quann, and G. D. Miller. 2013. "Meeting and Exceeding Dairy Recommendations: Effects of Dairy Consumption on Nutrient Intakes and Risk of Chronic Disease." *Nutrition Reviews* 71(4): 209–223.

Ryff, C. D. 2014. "Psychological Well-Being Revisited: Advances in the Science and Practice of Eudaimonia." *Psychotherapy and Psychosomatics* 83(1): 10–28.

Sachs, G. 2004. *Managing Bipolar Affective Disorder*. London: Science.

Scott, J., B. Stanton, A. Garland, and I. N. Ferrier. 2000. "Cognitive Vulnerability in Patients with Bipolar Disorder." *Psychological Medicine* 30(2): 467–472.

Sheldon, C., and T. A. Wills. 1985. "Stress, Social Support, and the Buffering Hypothesis." *Psychological Bulletin* 98(2): 310–357.

Soreca, I., E. Frank, and D. J. Kupfer. 2009. "The Phenomenology of Bipolar Disorder: What Drives the High Rate of Medical Burden and Determines Long-Term Prognosis?" *Depression and Anxiety* 26(1): 73–82.

Stoner, L., K. R. Stoner, J. M. Young, and S. Fryer. 2012. "Preventing a Cardiovascular Disease Epidemic Among Indigenous Populations Through Lifestyle Changes." *International Journal of Preventive Medicine* 3(4): 230–240.

Sylvia, L. G., E. S. Friedman, J. H. Kocsis, E. E. Bernstein, B. D. Brody, G. Kinrys, et al. 2013. "Association of Exercise with Quality of Life and Mood Symptoms in a Comparative Effectiveness Study of Bipolar Disorder." *Journal of Affective Disorders* 151(2): 722–727.

Sylvia, L. G., A. A. Nierenberg, J. P. Strange, A. D. Peckham, and T. Deckersbach. 2011. "Development of an Integrated Psychosocial Treatment to Address the Medical Burden in Bipolar Disorder." *Journal of Psychiatric Practice* 17(3): 224–232.

Sylvia, L. G., A. T. Peters, T. Deckersbach, and A. A. Nierenberg. 2013. "Nutrient-Based Therapies for Bipolar Disorder: A Systematic Review." *Psychotherapy and Psychosomatics* 82(1): 10–19.

Sylvia, L. G., S. Salcedo, E. E. Bernstein, J. H. Baek, A. A. Nierenberg, and T. Deckersbach. 2013. "Nutrition, Exercise, and Wellness Treatment in Bipolar Disorder: Proof of Concept for a Consolidated Intervention." *International Journal of Bipolar Disorders* 1(1): 1–7.

US Department of Agriculture. 2014. "Food Groups." http://www.choosemyplate.gov /food-groups. Accessed May 22, 2014.

Wegner, M., I. Helmich, S. Machado, A. E. Nardi, O. Arias-Carrion, and H. Budde. 2014. "Effects of Exercise on Anxiety and Depression Disorders: Review of Meta-Analyses and Neurobiological Mechanisms." *CNS and Neurological Disorders Drug Targets* 13(6): 1002–1014.

Weinberg, L., A. Hasni, M. Shinohara, and A. Duarte. 2014. "A Single Bout of Resistance Exercise Can Enhance Episodic Memory Performance." *Acta Psychologica* 153: 13–19.

Willett, W. C. 2011. *Eat, Drink, and Be Healthy: The Harvard Medical School Guide to Healthy Eating*. New York: Simon and Schuster.

Wing, R. R., W. Lang, T. A. Wadden, M. Safford, W. C. Knowler, A. G. Bertoni, et al. 2011. "Benefits of Modest Weight Loss in Improving Cardiovascular Risk Factors in Overweight and Obese Individuals with Type 2 Diabetes." *Diabetes Care* 34(7): 1481–1486.

Wright, K., T. Armstrong, A. Taylor, and S. Dean. 2012. "'It's a Double Edged Sword': A Qualitative Analysis of the Experiences of Exercise Amongst People with Bipolar Disorder." *Journal of Affective Disorders* 136(3): 634–642.

Yang, P. Y., K. H. Ho, H. C. Chen, and M. Y. Chien. 2012. "Exercise Training Improves Sleep Quality in Middle-Aged and Older Adults with Sleep Problems: A Systematic Review." *Journal of Physiotherapy* 58(3): 157–163.

Yatham, L. N., S. H. Kennedy, C. O'Donovan, S. Parikh, G. MacQueen, R. McIntyre, et al. 2005. "Canadian Network for Mood and Anxiety Treatments (CANMAT) Guidelines for the Management of Patients with Bipolar Disorder: Consensus and Controversies." *Bipolar Disorders* 7(suppl 3): 5–69.

Zschucke, E., A. Heinz, and A. Ströhle. 2012. "Exercise and Physical Activity in the Therapy of Substance Use Disorders." *Scientific World Journal*. [Epub ahead of print.]

Louisa Grandin Sylvia, PhD, is associate director of psychology at the Massachusetts General Hospital Bipolar Clinic and Research Program, director of health and wellness at the Red Sox Foundation and Massachusetts General Hospital Home Base Program, and assistant professor at Harvard Medical School. She is a skilled cognitive behavioral therapist who develops psychosocial interventions for bipolar disorder and serious mental illness. She is currently examining the efficacy of a nutrition, exercise, and wellness therapy for bipolar disorder.

Foreword writer **Andrew A. Nierenberg, MD**, is director of the Bipolar Clinic and Research Program and associate director of the Depression Clinic and Research Program at Massachusetts General Hospital, and professor of psychiatry at Harvard Medical School. Dr. Nierenberg has published over 400 papers and has been listed among the Best Doctors in North America for the treatment of mood and anxiety disorders continuously since 1994. He received the Gerald L. Klerman Young Investigator Award from the National Depressive and Manic Depression Association, the Brain and Behavior Foundation Colvin Prize for outstanding achievement in mood disorders research, and was listed among the World's Most Influential Scientific Minds 2014 by Thomson Reuters for having the top 1% of literature citations in psychiatry/psychology worldwide.

FROM OUR PUBLISHER—

As the publisher at New Harbinger and a clinical psychologist since 1978, I know that emotional problems are best helped with evidence-based therapies. These are the treatments derived from scientific research (randomized controlled trials) that show what works. Whether these treatments are delivered by trained clinicians or found in a self-help book, they are designed to provide you with proven strategies to overcome your problem.

Therapies that aren't evidence-based—whether offered by clinicians or in books—are much less likely to help. In fact, therapies that aren't guided by science may not help you at all. That's why this New Harbinger book is based on scientific evidence that the treatment can relieve emotional pain.

This is important: if this book isn't enough, and you need the help of a skilled therapist, use the following resources to find a clinician trained in the evidence-based protocols appropriate for your problem.

Real help is available for the problems you have been struggling with. The skills you can learn from evidence-based therapies will change your life.

Matthew McKay, PhD
Publisher, New Harbinger Publications

**If you need a therapist, the following organization
can help you find a therapist trained in cognitive behavioral therapy (CBT).**

The Association for Behavioral & Cognitive Therapies (ABCT) Find-a-Therapist service offers a list of therapists schooled in CBT techniques. Therapists listed are licensed professionals who have met the membership requirements of ABCT and who have chosen to appear in the directory.
Please visit www.abct.org and click on *Find a Therapist*.

For additional support for patients, family, and friends, contact the following:

Depression and Bipolar Support Alliance (DBSA) **Visit www.dbsalliance.org**

Bipolar Happens **Visit www.bipolarhappens.com**

For more new harbinger books, visit www.newharbinger.com

MORE BOOKS *from*
NEW HARBINGER PUBLICATIONS

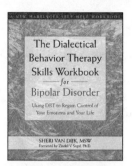

**THE DIALECTICAL
BEHAVIOR THERAPY SKILLS
WORKBOOK FOR
BIPOLAR DISORDER**

Using DBT to Regain Control of
Your Emotions & Your Life

ISBN: 978-1572246287 / US $21.95

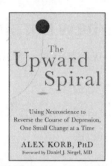

THE UPWARD SPIRAL

Using Neuroscience to Reverse
the Course of Depression,
One Small Change at a Time

ISBN: 978-1626251205 / US $16.95

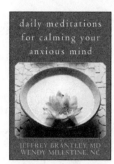

**DAILY MEDITATIONS
FOR CALMING YOUR
ANXIOUS MIND**

ISBN: 978-1572245402 / US $15.95

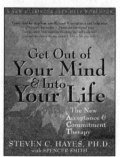

**GET OUT OF YOUR MIND
& INTO YOUR LIFE**

The New Acceptance &
Commitment Therapy

ISBN: 978-1572244252 / US $21.95

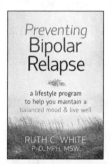

**PREVENTING BIPOLAR
RELAPSE**

A Lifestyle Program to Help
You Maintain a Balanced
Mood & Live Well

ISBN: 978-1608828814 / US $16.95

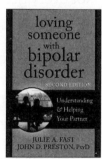

**LOVING SOMEONE
WITH BIPOLAR DISORDER,
SECOND EDITION**

Understanding & Helping
Your Partner

ISBN: 978-1608822195 / US $16.95

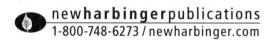

newharbingerpublications
1-800-748-6273 / newharbinger.com

(VISA, MC, AMEX / prices subject to change without notice)

Like us on Facebook: facebook.com/newharbinger   Follow us on Twitter: @newharbinger.com

Don't miss out on new books in the subjects that interest you.
Sign up for our **Book Alerts** at **newharbinger.com/bookalerts**

Register your **new harbinger** titles for additional benefits!

When you register your **new harbinger** title—purchased in any format, from any source—you get access to benefits like the following:

- Downloadable accessories like printable worksheets and extra content

- Instructional videos and audio files

- Information about updates, corrections, and new editions

Not every title has accessories, but we're adding new material all the time.

Access free accessories in 3 easy steps:

1. Sign in at NewHarbinger.com (or **register** to create an account).

2. Click on **register a book**. Search for your title and click the **register** button when it appears.

3. Click on the **book cover or title** to go to its details page. Click on **accessories** to view and access files.

That's all there is to it!

If you need help, visit:

NewHarbinger.com/accessories

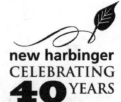

new harbinger
CELEBRATING
40 YEARS